Quality care for elderly people

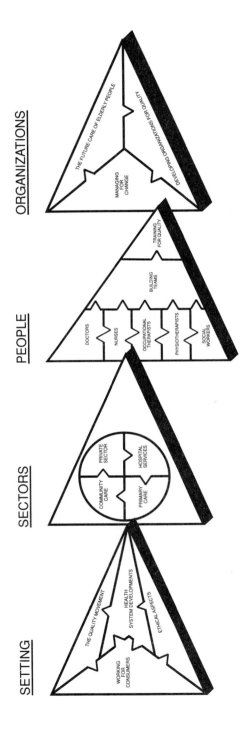

Quality care for elderly people

Edited by

Peter P. Mayer MA FRCP
Institute of Ageing and Health, Moseley Hall Hospital
Birmingham, UK

Edward J. Dickinson
MA MBA FRCP
Royal College of Physicians Research Unit, London, UK

and

Martin Sandler MB ChB MRCP
Department of Geriatric Medicine, Solihull Hospital
West Midlands, UK

CHAPMAN & HALL MEDICAL

London · Weinheim · New York · Tokyo · Melbourne · Madras

Published by Chapman & Hall,
2–6 Boundary Row, London SE1 8HN, UK

Chapman & Hall, 2–6 Boundary Row, London SE1 8HN, UK

Chapman & Hall GmbH, Pappelallee 3, 69469 Weinheim, Germany

Chapman & Hall USA, Fourth Floor, 115 Fifth Avenue, New York
NY 10003, USA

Chapman & Hall Japan, ITP-Japan, Kyowa Building, 3F, 2-2-1 Hirakawacho,
Chiyoda-ku, Tokyo 102, Japan

DA Book (Aust.) Pty Ltd, 648 Whitehorse Road, Mitcham 3132, Victoria,
Australia

Chapman & Hall India, R. Seshadri, 32 Second Main Road, CIT East,
Madras 600 035, India

First edition 1997

© 1997 Chapman & Hall

Typeset in 10/12pt Centennial by Best-Set Typesetters, Hong Kong

Printed in Great Britain by Alden Press, Oxford

ISBN 0 412 61830 3

A catalogue record for this book is available from the British Library

Library of Congress Catalog Card Number: 96–83762

 Printed on acid free text paper, manufactured in accordance with ANSI/NISO
Z39.48-1992 (Permanence of Paper)

Contents

Contributors

Richard Baker MB FRCGP
Director
Eli Lilly National Clinical Audit Centre
Department of General Practice and Primary Health Care
University of Leicester
Leicester, UK

Carole Brown BA MBA MCSP SRP
Disability Services Manager
Community Health Care Service (North Derbyshire) NHS Trust
Chesterfield, UK

David Challis BA MSc CertPSW CertEd PhD
Professor of Social Work and Community Care
Personal Social Services Research Unit
University of Kent at Canterbury
Canterbury, UK

Terry Devenney FFA
Director
Devenney-Wilkes Management Services Ltd
Birmingham, UK

Edward J. Dickinson MA MBA FRCP
Associate Director
Royal College of Physicians Research Unit
London, UK

Fleur Fisher
Formerly Head of Ethics, Science and Information Division
British Medical Association
London, UK

Christine A. Graham Dip COT SROT SP DipA MISPA
Consultant Occupational Therapist and Aromatherapist
Walsall, UK

Sally Greengross OBE
Director General
Age Concern
London, UK

Ann Hunter MA FCSP
Project Manager
Centre for Medical Education
University of Dundee
Dundee, UK

Tom Keighley RGN RMN NDNCert RCNT
DN (Lond) BA(Hons)
Director, International Development
School of Health Care Studies
University of Leeds
Leeds, UK

Barbara Laing MSocSC CQSW DipSW
Regional General Manager (West Midlands)
Anchor Trust
Birmingham, UK

Karen A. Luker PhD BNurs RGN RHV NDNCert
Director
Department of Nursing
Research and Development Unit
University of Liverpool
Liverpool, UK

Steven Luttrell BSc (Hons) MB ChB MRCP
Dip (Law) Barrister
Senior Registrar
Department of Geriatric Medicine
Whittington Hospital
London, UK

Peter P. Mayer MA FRCP
The Institute of Ageing and Health (West Midlands)
Moseley Hall Hospital
Birmingham, UK

Peter H. Millard MD FRCP
Eleanor Peel Professor of Geriatric Medicine
Division of Geriatric Medicine
St George's Hospital Medical School
London, UK

Pennie Roberts MCSP
Disability Services Manager
Community Health Care Service (North Derbyshire)
NHS Trust
Chesterfield, UK

David L. Sandler MB ChB MRCP
Senior Registrar in Geriatric Medicine
Birmingham Heartlands Hospital
Birmingham, UK

Martin Sandler MB ChB MRCP
Consultant Physician
Solihull Hospital
Solihull, UK

Elizabeth M. Smith MB ChB MRCP
Consultant in Geriatric Medicine
Sandwell Hospital
Birmingham, UK

Peter S. Stansbie ACIS MHSM MMS DMS
Chief Executive
Dyfed Powys Health Authority
St David's Hospital
Carmarthen, UK

Gillian B. Todd MB BCh FFPHM
Chief Executive
Bro Taf Health Authority
Cardiff, UK

Philip Tormey
Devenney-Wilkes Management Services Ltd
Birmingham, UK

Karen Traske BA MA
Research Officer
Personal Social Services Unit
University of Kent at Canterbury
Canterbury, UK

Karen R. Waters
Senior Lecturer in Nursing
School of Nursing Studies
University of Manchester
Manchester, UK

Preface

This book is all about improving the health care of elderly people, which is facing unprecedented challenges in the 1990s. Energies need to be concentrated in three main areas:

- the development of high quality care in community settings
- the future role of specialized hospital services
- the way that long-term care is delivered.

All of these are interconnected and success with any of them depends on successful relationships. For example, success in community care requires working interfaces with primary care, the private sector and hospital care. These interfaces are not static but comprise dynamic interactions between people – people in different teams, with different backgrounds, training, perspectives and interests. What people do is influenced strongly by the organizations they work for.

These inescapable facts lead us to the structure of this book. By concentrating on sectors, people and organizations, we hope to deal with all the important relationships in a coherent way. Yet this book is not intended to be from a service providers' perspective. We have arranged the book in this way so that providers are best equipped to meet the needs of their customers – whether they are patients, residents or clients. We know that elderly people may experience dislocation in their care because of frictions and gaps between different sectors, disciplines, teams and organizations. To achieve seamless care, there is a need for greater understanding and harmony of purpose and action across the care spectrum.

The aim of this book is to assist all those who have an interest, role or responsibility in developing high quality care. Reflecting this, the contributors to this book make up an expert team and their diversity indicates the need for teamwork in service development. This is a practical book that has been written largely by people with direct experience. However, most of the book is underpinned by the theory that provides readers with principles and frameworks. We hope readers will find the book relevant to the present, in a rapidly changing area.

How should the reader approach this book? We recommend that everyone reads Part One, which provides settings, because this emphasizes the consumer approach that is required in developing high quality services. In Part Two, which looks at sectors, it may be most useful to concentrate on sectors other than your own. The same applies to the different disciplines covered in Part Three, but team building and training will be relevant to most. Although Part Four, on organizations, may look as if it is for managers, remember that we all work within organizations. This part is relevant to all those concerned with the care of elderly people – manager or not – concentrating as it does on change, quality and the future.

You can read the book from beginning to end and the editors' introductions to each chapter provide continuity. Alternatively, the book can be dipped into at will as each chapter stands alone. Indeed, we have deliberately retained the individual style and approach of each contributor.

The four parts of this book are intended to provide four interconnected slices across care.

- **Part One Setting** This part is concerned with the wider environment within which services are organized and care is delivered. The book opens with a chapter that has a consumer focus, indicating the needs of patients and their families in shaping services. Chapter 2 builds on this perspective by considering how ethical issues have a central role in influencing care delivery. This is followed by two complementary chapters which paint the political and quality management backdrop for the book. Chapter 3 explains recent developments in the health system, while Chapter 4 describes the relationship between quality in health services and other sectors.
- **Part Two Sectors** This part uncovers the contribution of the different sectors of care and explores quality initiatives in each. We begin, in Chapter 5, with primary care and progress through community care (Chapter 6), private sector care (Chapter 7) and hospital care (Chapter 8). The importance of this part is that those developing high quality health care need to consider the interfaces and relationships between the different sectors. In this way one can respond to the need to re-engineer different aspects of the process of care in different sectors.
- **Part Three People** This part recognizes that high quality care is fundamentally dependent on people, and examines

the issue in two ways. First, the contributions of some of the different care disciplines are discussed in Chapter 9. This is followed by an analysis of how to build effective teams (Chapter 10). This part ends with a wider perspective on the role of training in developing staff who are competent to deliver high quality care (Chapter 11).

- **Part Four Organizations** This part aims to put the previous considerations into the context of organizations for care and how they can respond to the future. Chapter 12 deals with the general issue of managing change which will be relevant to any quality initiative. Chapter 13 widens out the discussion to evaluate how quality can become a core part of services. The book closes with an analysis of future developments (Chapter 14).

This book contains devices to assist the reader in using it to best effect.

- **Book at a glance** The whole book is shown diagrammatically in the frontispiece and the components of each part are similarly shown at the beginning of each part.
- **Editors' introductions** Each chapter begins with an Editors' Introduction which outlines the main focus of the chapter, identifies key topics and indicates connections with other chapters.
- **Essential points** Every chapter can be scanned quickly using the essential points in the margin, which also specifically indicate quality examples and practice points.

After reading the book you will have gained three interlinked benefits. First, you will have an excellent overview of all aspects of the high quality care of elderly people as told by acknowledged experts in the field. Second, this will be backed up with access to practical advice on how to improve matters. Finally, you will be equipped with the relevant theoretical knowledge both to make sense of what is going on around you, and to participate in discussions with those you wish to influence.

Peter P. Mayer, Edward J. Dickinson and Martin Sandler
Birmingham and London, UK

Acknowledgements

The editors would like to thank four main groups of people who made this book possible.

- **Contributors** We are grateful to all the contributors who agreed to participate in this interdisciplinary book.
- **Publishers** We could not have managed without the editorial staff of Chapman & Hall who gave invaluable guidance and advice.
- **Colleagues** We are indebted to our long-suffering colleagues and secretaries who put up with our preoccupied demeanour during the preparation of this book.
- **Family** Finally, the biggest thank-you goes to our families who provided unstinting support throughout.

Part One
Setting

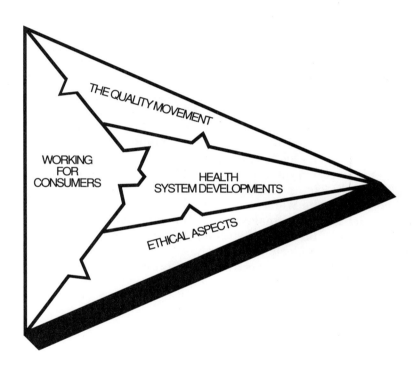

THE QUALITY MOVEMENT

WORKING
FOR
CONSUMERS

HEALTH
SYSTEM DEVELOPMENTS

ETHICAL ASPECTS

EDITORS' INTRODUCTION TO PART ONE

The health care of elderly people takes place in an ever changing environment. Political, social, economic and technological changes may all affect what is provided, how it is provided and where it is provided. This means that developing high quality health care must take into account what is going on outside disciplines, specialties, services and sectors.

The purpose of Part One is to provide a snapshot of what is going on in the present environment by drawing out and illustrating the main issues. To do this three main themes are explored:

- consumerism
- health service reorganization
- the quality revolution.

Chapter 1, 'Working for consumers', sets the scene for the rapid trend towards patient-centred services by describing in detail what consumers need from services in the context of the main service changes that are occurring.

Chapter 2, 'Ethical aspects of the quality of care', develops the consumerist theme further by discussing quality at the level of individual decisions. This is done within the framework of ethics and provides a powerful rationale for putting the patient first.

Chapter 3, 'Recent health system developments', introduces the effects of the health service reorganization. By looking at commissioning, trusts, GP fundholding and community care, links are made between quality and changing structures, functions and relationships.

Chapter 4, 'The quality movement', places the development of high quality services within the context of the wider quality revolution in services. The concept of the quality toolbox is introduced to try and make sense of the myriad of quality activities that may be encountered.

By the end of this part, the reader will be aware of the key external issues in relation to high quality care for elderly people. These will surface and resurface throughout the book, being examined from the perspectives of different sectors and disciplines involved in care.

Working for consumers 1

Sally Greengross

EDITORS' INTRODUCTION

This opening chapter deliberately looks at care from the perspective of the consumer. Although in the past many services, especially public services, have been more orientated to the provider, major changes are now occurring. Lady Greengross initiates major themes that will reccur throughout the book and are reinforced by the subsequent chapter on ethical approaches to care.

This chapter is made up of seven main parts. First, the challenges to excellent care are elucidated; these range from the philosophical to the practical and present a menu of issues that need solutions. Next, the dramatic alteration to the perspectives of the consumer is described. This is multifactorial in origin but highlights the need to fuse the agendas of consumers and providers. This is followed by an important section on protecting older people's interests at the individual, sector and service levels, particularly within the context of service fragmentation. A special look is given to both the new development of community-based care schemes and the challenges of long-term care, with a special focus on funding. The influence of economic circumstances and education is introduced in the positive context of health promotion. The distinctive role of the voluntary sector is explained using practical examples. Finally, the future is analysed by discussing how success should be measured and which principles should be followed.

After reading this chapter, you will have a broad feel for the key issues, particularly those that are practical and political. This chapter describes an extensive range of areas for debate and development in relation to consumerism in the care of

Key topics
- Challenges
- Switch to consumerism
- Protecting older people's interests
- Caring in the community
- Future long-term care
- Health promotion
- Role of the voluntary sector
- Facing the future

Quality Care for Elderly People. Edited by Peter P. Mayer, Edward J. Dickinson and Martin Sandler. Published in 1997 by Chapman & Hall, London. ISBN 0 412 61830 3

older people. To develop the specific theme of consumerism, you should consult:

- the subsequent chapter, which details practical approaches to empowering individuals in the context of illness;
- Chapter 4, which considers the role of consumerism in the quality movement.

CHALLENGES TO EXCELLENT CARE

Challenges
- Longevity
- Philosophy
- Care demarcations
- Patient empowerment
- Ageism
- Long-term care
- Care costs

The dramatic increase in the number of older people in this country is well documented. Yet the number of carers, as we know them today, is predicted to drop sharply as the ratio of middle-aged women to very old people falls and as more women of this age group work, 77% estimated for 2001 compared with 62% in 1971. The proportion of older people living alone is also increasing: it is estimated that by 2001 there will be a net increase of over 600 000 compared with 1986. The significance for service providers is that living alone is the highest risk factor, after age itself, for admission to hospital or to long-term care.

The then Secretary of State for Health, Virginia Bottomley, writing in the *Independent* in August 1994, reflected the concern of many:

> In the NHS today the question is how we can best continue to provide a cradle to grave medical service to an ageing population whose longevity we are working hard to enhance.

Older people are major consumers of care services, the demarcation of which into acute, chronic, health and social care is often meaningless when applied to an age cohort that extends across 30 years or more and is composed of people who often present with multiple pathologies.

Few would argue with the concept that older people should receive the care they need and that they should be empowered whenever possible to make decisions about that care. For this to happen they must be fully aware of the real choices available, both for care and for treatment, so that their decisions are genuinely informed. The goal must be to use to the full their capacity to understand sufficiently the implication of any decisions they make.

We know that many older people's expectations, already tending to be lower than those of younger people, are likely to be further reduced as they age. Similarly, a degree of impairment, which earlier they might have found unacceptable, may be tolerated later on, but for older people to be made to feel a burden on the NHS is not acceptable, especially when they are frequently told by the media that the older generation has never been as fit as it is today. Unfortunately there is still a widespread belief that people who do not have very long to live should not receive expensive medical intervention, regardless of the extent to which it might enhance the quality of the life they have left.

The shift to a policy of care in the community is an explicitly declared commitment to meeting the diverse and multiple needs of older people. Structuring services on the basis of assessed needs, and giving older people and their carers a say in decision making, increases choice and enables people to stay in their own homes wherever possible. However, the enthusiastic pursual of a policy to keep people at home may well result in particular difficulties being experienced by those who do need continuing care elsewhere than at home; while their numbers are small at present, the projected growth in the older population overall will mean that the number of those in need of long-term care will increase quite significantly in the foreseeable future.

The escalating costs of care are also a key factor affecting current policy. The so-called 'perverse incentive', which encouraged service providers in the 1980s to seek residential care, largely paid for by government funds, led to an unprecedented boom in private sector homes and is also manifest in health care provision. However, if cost-containment becomes the main reason for the provision of a particular type of service, this will lead to poor care and, in the long term, may well result in higher costs to deal with the unforeseen consequences of such a short-sighted approach.

> **Practice point**
> Short-term cost-containment
> • can lead to poor care
> • may result in higher overall costs

THE SWITCH TO CONSUMERISM

The voting strength of older people is now beginning to be recognized and there is a general awareness of the increasing economic importance of the older age group. The wealth of some older people has led to targeted health care products, following the trend previously evident in, for example, the leisure, lifestyle opportunities and travel sectors. However, the majority of older people still depend on the basic State pension for most of their income, and for them means-tested

> **Sources of consumerism**
> • Voting strength
> • Economic importance
> • Patient's Charter
> • Involving people in choices

care can be extremely problematic, when they may already be experiencing difficulties in making ends meet.

This generation had expectations of cradle to grave health care, provided and funded by the NHS through a welfare state that would look after all their health needs. They can no more distinguish between social care and health care, than can most other people, particularly as the needs of older people will often vacillate between the two as their health improves or gets worse.

The Patient's Charter gives people the right to complain and, in certain cases, to make a claim for compensation if standards are not met. This is just one factor that has raised people's expectations, perhaps unrealistically in current circumstances. However, having raised expectations, something needs to be done about meeting them. Although laudable, the principle that excellent care should be achieved by involving users in both definition and determination of quality is, in reality, ahead of practice. There is little evidence as yet of consumers being involved in, for example, setting contract specifications, although growing importance is being attached to consumer feedback in monitoring services.

We need to concentrate on the most effective ways of talking with, and listening to, users of services. Group meetings may be dominated by those who are more vociferous and may therefore become unrepresentative. Questionnaires do not always work; many consumers find them alien, and inappropriate design may result in not achieving a correct response. Older people, perhaps more than other groups, demonstrate a sense of gratitude that may inhibit frank feedback, so time is needed to involve them fully along with encouragement if they are to make suggestions for improvements or perhaps participate in focus groups. Sensitive approaches to meet the needs of people for whom spoken English, vision or hearing present difficulties are important, as is transport, which can be the main factor deterring people from being involved. They also need to see results and to feel that their input is acted upon.

A balance must be struck between professional and consumer definitions of quality. The philosophy underlying good day care in the eyes of the professional might include a more protective environment, whereas the consumer may see it in terms of social enjoyment and participation. Sometimes consumers can be unrealistic, and professionals can be reluctant to give up entrenched positions, but in reality assumptions may be different, albeit equally valid.

Challenges in user involvement
- Unrepresentativeness
- Alien questionnaires
- Time
- Communication barriers
- Professional definitions of quality

We need to remember that quality is related to resources and rationing, and that the choice may be between a high quality service for a few or a lower quality service for many. Consumers are, on the whole, able to understand this dichotomy and, if they are part of the discussion, offer a valuable perspective. We need to know what they see as essential and what they feel to be less of a priority. By listening to them, we may find that we use our resources better. One positive trend is the increasing number of advocacy services through which more account is given to the needs of carers, who can now expect a separate assessment of their particular needs. This is important as these can be different from those of the people for whom they are caring.

PROTECTING OLDER PEOPLE'S INTERESTS

Any treatment must be based on the individual's diagnosis, prognosis and assessment of care needs, and include rehabilitation and the time to recover fully. Excellent care must not group patients into categories based on their chronological age. This is an inherently discriminatory practice and grossly unfair.

Care packages must be accessible geographically and presented in a meaningful and comprehensible way. Older people must receive a standard of care that does not vary according to the area in which they live.

A clear definition is needed of the boundaries between health and social care to avoid expectations being dashed, e.g. through the fear of being unable to pay for services which they had assumed would be funded by the NHS.

Joint commissioning may be the most promising way forward in the longer term to ensure that older people do not suffer. However, some sorting out is essential immediately, or else the divide between health and social care will undermine the potential for excellent care that recent policies were intended to facilitate, as the argument shifts to primarily one of who pays for which type of service.

The profusion of change in the provision of both health and care demands special vigilance if the interests of older people are to be protected. A full range of health services is needed in each area if excellent care is to be a reality. Older people need to remain near their homes as they are often very dependent on a declining number of close relatives or friends for visitors, who may themselves have difficulty in travelling far.

Key pathways
- Avoid ageism
- Access fairness
- Clarify health and social care boundary
- Joint commissioning
- Comprehensive local specialized services

Principles
Services should be:
- local
- comprehensive
- appropriately staffed

Some tasks previously carried out by nursing staff are now done by home carers. Consequently, the boundary between nursing and care assistance is more difficult to define, and some tasks previously taken for granted may not be carried out at all. Nursing home staff are now doing some work that was previously carried out in hospitals, and there may be increased dependency levels among older people remaining at home, with too few and often overstretched domiciliary care staff being asked to take on tasks for which they have had little or no training, such as changing catheters. In future such difficulties may increase as the costs of care continue to rise and the contribution of the NHS diminishes. Guidance issued by the Department of Health in February 1995 recognized that some health authorities may have gone too far in reducing their continuing care beds, action that has far reaching consequences on other services, which are rapidly becoming stretched to capacity.

Assessment of people's needs by local authorities is a requirement of the NHS and Community Care Act, 1990, but having to meet these needs within available resources can lead to wide local variations and budget-led decisions, which in turn tends to focus attention on the most frail at the expense of basic prevention and support services.

Now that residential and nursing home care requires means-testing, fundamental questions are raised. Many older people face a lack of availability of NHS dentistry, physiotherapy, occupational and speech therapy, and chiropody. Even basic nail cutting services are scarce, and bathing is a particularly difficult issue, partly because there is a need to resolve whether this is a health or a social service. Unfortunately, the withdrawal of fully funded services that are disproportionately needed by older people is likely to increase because of the worry about who will pay.

Threats
- Service variations
- Budget primacy
- Emphasis on frailty
- Scarce vital services

CARING IN THE COMMUNITY

Some of the new provisions in both health and social care in the community have undoubtedly been a success, and the speed of change in their implementation has been most impressive. Nevertheless, while there may be more sensitivity to the needs of the consumers of health care and more people are being treated, older people are often the last to benefit and some of the perceived gains do not appear to be getting through to them.

Although the cost of caring for someone at home is high, over a long period it may well be cheaper than caring for that person in a residential or nursing home, and staying at home is certainly what most older people say they want. This means a major switch is needed to provide outreach care, possibly involving all sectors. For example, many more residential and nursing homes could increase their provision of domiciliary care and extend their facilities to include more rehabilitation.

One dilemma relates to hospital discharge procedures. Research on this by the Royal College of General Practitioners showed there are fewer people using beds inappropriately and there is a reduction in the time patients have to wait to leave hospital. Fast throughput may be excellent for younger patients, and is good in theory for everyone, but it can be unfortunate for many older people who need longer to recover from invasive treatment. If they are discharged too early from hospital, the result can be readmission at a later stage with a more grave outcome.

Excellent care must cover a full assessment of people's care needs with convalescence and rehabilitation built in, rather than being limited to concentrating on discharge home or to a long-term stay in hospital, thus adding to the perceived problem of bed-blocking. It is unfortunate that older people seem to be blamed as though they were responsible for inadequate or wrongly allocated resources.

> **Dilemmas**
> - The cost of developing long-term home care services
> - Speeding up hospital discharge
> - The need for rehabilitation

THE FUTURE FOR LONG-TERM CARE

Long-term health care services are declining as the number of older people increases. There is a question mark over whether the NHS will provide sufficient high quality care in the future. Laing and Buisson (1995) estimate that 75 000 places were provided in 1970, whereas by 1994 there were only 54 800. The number of local authority residential homes has also been much reduced; only in the independent sector has there been growth in the number of both residential and nursing homes.

The funding of long-term care concerns many people in a fast changing world. The future of a welfare state in which people pay when they are working and receive care when they need it, is now no longer certain. A shift towards personal responsibility for paying for care reflects the government's attitude to funding, and the decline in NHS long-term provision is part of that policy shift.

One possible way forward might be to follow the example of Germany, which recently introduced compulsory insurance, paid by all employees with a matching contribution from employers: a hypothecated tax to pay exclusively for long-term care.

The UK government is now considering several options that could lead to individuals being required to meet all or part of their long-term care costs in the future. This is causing a lot of anxiety at a time when rapid changes in the labour market and increased uncertainty about jobs and occupational pensions make the ability of people to pay for their own continuing health care less rather than more likely.

Whether long-term care is received in independent residential or nursing homes or through the NHS, both needs and costs are rising fast. Laing and Buisson (1995) estimate that 72 000 more places will be needed by the end of the century to meet the increased number of people aged 85 years and over, who represent the highest proportion of people in need of long-term care. Excellent care must include preventive measures and more emphasis on the maintenance of good health, otherwise in the future people may live longer but not in better health, rather in a state of increased dependency.

HEALTH PROMOTION – A HOLISTIC APPROACH

Action areas
- Poverty
- Education
- Screening

To meet needs, adequate care provision must take account of social and financial circumstances. Poverty may render people less capable of caring for themselves; those living in more privileged circumstances have fewer illnesses and live longer than the more deprived. Death rates are two to three times higher in low, compared with high, socioeconomic groups. Such differences are key contributors to most causes of death, and together they reduce the life expectancy of the least privileged by some eight years.

Much discomfort and illness among older people could be alleviated by sound education, regular health checks and more sensible lifestyles. Every year, 100 000 people in the UK experience a first stroke. This is a major problem, with only a small proportion of victims ever regaining full use of their faculties.

Recent controversy over the age limit for automatic invitations to breast screening for women aged 65+ is an example of a cost-effective method of keeping people healthy which at present is subject to age discriminatory practice. In addition, osteoporosis, leading to about 43 000 hip fractures annually in the UK, might be reduced if more older women were offered the choice of hormone replacement therapy (HRT) and other preventive measures.

The World Health Organization views good health as total well-being. This especially emphasizes that to be in good health in later life means using one's faculties and capacities as fully as possible, even if some deterioration has taken place. Older people who remain involved in their community and who retain strong family links are likely to live longer and be happier. This reinforces the importance of the higher profile the UK Government is now giving to health promotion and the prevention of disease through the Health of the Nation initiative. That older people were not singled out for special treatment in this is a matter of some regret; however, most of the current health targets apply to them. The danger is always that they will be left behind while other groups are treated as a priority. The value and potential health gain in focusing on older people should not be underestimated.

One example of what can be done is 'Ageing Well', a major initiative co-ordinated by Age Concern England in the UK and in partnership across Europe. Piloted in several areas within the UK, its aim is to improve and maintain the health of older people and prevent disease through a multisectoral and multidisciplinary approach.

Closely tied to the Health of the Nation targets, it depends very largely on the resource provided by older people themselves as 'senior health mentors'. They support other older people and act as advisers and friends. People they work with may find someone of their own age and background easier to speak to in confidence. Through giving older people the opportunity to practise what they want to say to their family doctor, the cost-effectiveness of the time spent with the GP and compliance with his or her prescriptions or treatment may well be improved. Senior health mentors can get across simple but very effective messages, such as the value of healthy eating. Simple changes in diet and regular exercise can achieve spectacular improvement in health, but many people are unaware of how quickly and effectively this can happen.

This initiative meets one of the most important aims of organizations like Age Concern, which works closely with

> **Quality example**
> Ageing Well:
> - Partnership
> - Mentors

older people and demonstrates that this age group can be active and contribute much to society.

THE ROLE OF THE VOLUNTARY SECTOR

As a service provider in a plural system of welfare the voluntary sector is a factor that increases choice. Having their own distinct character, voluntary organizations take a different and often innovative and pioneering approach, seeking new ways of meeting needs. At their best, voluntary organizations offer services within a community, provided by the community, working together with the group they seek to serve. Many are now entering into formal contractual relationships, providing what purchasers want at affordable costs. Consequently, the voluntary sector has to become both more accountable and professional to ensure and maintain better standards. One risk in taking on this new role could be a loss of spontaneity, inhibiting the outspokenness of voluntary organizations, and, as service providers, making them less willing to campaign. It would be sad if the constructively critical role and the innovative potential of the voluntary sector are in any way diminished by voluntary bodies shifting their accountability towards the purchaser instead of continuing to see their users as their first priority. The ethical relationship must remain primarily with the consumer, otherwise there is a risk that the character of services could change.

Setting standards for care

Voluntary organizations working in the field of community care are well placed to help set and monitor standards. Many have as their aim the provision of as friendly an environment as possible for their day centres. However, within such an environment, people's rights and responsibilities as users need to be clearly identified, giving them as much choice as possible in determining what services are available, how and when people are transported to and from the day centre, and extending to chairing and holding meetings without staff if that is their wish. Users also have responsibilities to respect the rights of other users, staff and volunteers. As well as setting standards for its day care, Age Concern has drawn up comprehensive descriptions and 'conditions of service' for clients who receive its services in their own homes, so that they know exactly what to expect and what is expected of

Practice point
Contracts increase:
• accountability
• professionalism

Contracts may reduce:
• spontaneity
• advocacy

Practice point
Consumer-based standards in day centres

them. Items include advocacy, translating and interpreting services, insurance and complaints procedures.

Residential care

Regardless of which sector is the provider, the interests of residents, as well as those of the providing organization, should be fairly reflected in any contract. Anyone looking at this form of care for the first time can find it a bewildering and frightening experience, and checklists can help to guide them through it. These can cover, among other areas, agreement on fees, levels of care, facilities, recreational activities, times, places and choices regarding meals, personal furnishings and possessions, GP and medication arrangements and many more items, including policy on pets.

Contracts should be even-handed and respect the rights of residents, outlining the circumstances in which they may be asked to leave because of a deterioration in their condition, or for other reasons, but the contract should stipulate a reasonable notice period of perhaps six weeks, and provide access to help in finding more suitable accommodation. Most importantly, the contract should ensure that no one be required to leave until alternative accommodation is found.

> **Practice point**
> A checklist can be useful when making residential care choices

> **Practice point**
> Contracts should offer reasonable protection

FACING THE FUTURE – ENSURING EXCELLENCE

It is important to measure success if we are to provide excellent care. This may be in terms of improvements in people's quality of life, increased choice, or increased control over people's lifestyle and environment. It may mean taking account of people who are losing out through the changes as well as those who are experiencing better care, e.g. those who no longer receive services because they are now not considered to be frail enough or sufficiently at risk.

The satisfaction level of consumers of services must also be sought. We want to know whether the wider choice of providers and care options available is real and whether providers are more responsive to the needs of the users of these services. Are care packages flexible and related to real needs and outcomes, or are they budget-led? Is the care provided as a seamless service to the consumer, or are the gaps and delays no better than previously? All those involved must work in partnership to ensure that users, whether older people or their carers, are consulted, take part in the

> **Measuring success**
> • Quality of life
> • Choice and Control
> • Satisfaction
> • Seamlessness
> • Consumer focus

planning process and have an opportunity to give their opinions on the type of care they are receiving and on the management process supporting its delivery.

We have to ensure that excellent care is available for people who need it today, otherwise we deny them the benefits of a long-standing obligation and fail to fulfil the expectations of those who pioneered and, in their view, paid for a system of welfare for everyone. To ensure excellent care for older people will require a commitment and determination to work together by people from many disciplines and sectors: policy makers as well as practitioners, those who plan as well as those who implement, and, above all, older people themselves, who must feel they are individuals of worth and value and that they are cared about, as well as for, in the years ahead.

> **Principles for success**
> • Putting consumers first
> • Working together
> • Involvement across the full spectrum of care

FURTHER READING

Schneidawind, D. (1994) *Long term Insurance in Germany*, available from Münchener Rückversicherungs-Gesellschaft, Königinstrasse 107, D-80791 München, Germany.

'*Ageing Well*' publications
(1994) *Helping Yourself to Health: Health Sessions with Older People: A 'How To' Guide*, Age Concern England, London.
(1994) *Health Promotion with Older People: Ideas for Primary Health Care Teams*, Age Concern England, London.
Nash, C. and Carter, T. (1994) *The Age Well Handbook: Setting Up of Community Health Initiatives with Older People*, Age Concern England, London.
(1993) *Age Well Planning and Ideas Pack*, Age Concern England, London.
(1995) *Inquiry into Long-Term Care – Evidence to the Health Select Committee 1995. NHS Responsibilities for Continuing Health Care, and Hospital Discharge Arrangements*, Age Concern England, London.
(1995) *Comments on the Department of the Environment's Consultation Paper 'Deregulating Local Government: The First Steps'*, Age Concern England, London.
(1995) *Comments to the Department of Health on Draft Guidance on Community Care Plans for 1996/97 in England*, Age Concern England, London.
(1995) *Moving the Goalposts: Changing Policies for Long-Stay Health and Social Care of Elderly People*, Age Concern England, London.

Age Concern Contracts Unit (1993) *Community Care: Agreement with Users*, Age Concern, London.

Laing, W. (1993) *Financing Long Term Care*, ACE Books.

Laing and Buisson (1995) *Care of Elderly People: Market Survey*, Laing and Buisson, London.

McLone, F. and Cronin, N. (1994) *A Crisis in Care? The future of family and State care for older people in the European Union*, Family Policy Studies Centre and Centre for Policy on Ageing, London.

Society and Health (1994) Centre for Health and Society at University College London and the King's Fund Institute.

Ethical aspects of quality care 2

Steven Luttrell and Fleur Fisher

EDITORS' INTRODUCTION

This chapter expands on the previous one by dealing with practical aspects of the quality of individual care using the principles of ethics. Although ethics are regarded as rather a 'dry' subject by some, this chapter brings the theory alive and is full of practical advice on how to base excellent care on ethical care.

This chapter is made up of five main parts. Autonomy is a word that is widely used. The authors define it, explain its legal basis and consider the relationship between old age, frailty and autonomy. Next, capacity is tackled, with practical advice on how to assess it and how to improve it. Autonomy may, wrongly, be assumed to be diminished among elderly people. There is an underlying assumption that capacity to make decisions exists until proved otherwise. Elderly people face two difficulties here. First, the opposite assumption may be made. Second, elderly people commonly experience health problems that threaten their capacity. Practical advice for improving capacity and empowering elderly patients is given, along with a checklist for informal planning to assist later decision making. In contrast, more formal mechanisms may be required when decision making capacity is lost. This leads to the third main topic – advance directives. These are discussed in relation to the Enduring Power of Attorney and informal recording of patients' wishes, and the American experience, with advice on how to discuss this difficult area with elderly people.

Fourth, euthanasia is discussed with an international perspective, leading to a wide consideration of rationing, which is the final topic. Rationing is a highly emotive topic

Key topics
- Autonomy
- Capacity
- Advance directives
- Euthanasia
- Rationing

Quality Care for Elderly People. Edited by Peter P. Mayer, Edward J. Dickinson and Martin Sandler. Published in 1997 by Chapman & Hall, London. ISBN 0 412 61830 3

but it is tackled in a reasoned and illuminating fashion by considering various rationing approaches. In order to ensure equity and justice more information is required about costs and outcomes to allow rationing by utility. To take these themes forward will require partnership between patients, carers, providers of all disciplines, purchasers and policy makers.

After reading this chapter, you will have an excellent grasp of how ethics can be used as a basis for delivering high quality care. This chapter examines ethical aspects of high quality care in depth, providing clear explanations and practical tools to use in common day to day situations. What is discussed is certainly relevant to all sectors and all disciplines. Readers may find they need to refer back to this chapter when reading about community care and hospital care in particular.

INTRODUCTION

A quality care system is one that is concerned with improving clinical outcome, efficiency and patient satisfaction. Autonomy and justice are two fundamental ethical principles that should lie at the heart of any quality care system. Every person has a right to self-determination and any method for rationing health care should be equitable.

AUTONOMY

'The right to determine what shall be done with one's own body is a fundamental right in our society. The concepts inherent in this right are the bedrock upon which principles of self-determination and individual autonomy are based. Free individual choice in matters affecting this should, in my opinion, be accorded very high priority . . .'
(Robins JA, *Malette* v. *Schulman*, 1990)

Under English law (and the laws of many other jurisdictions), the doctor has a duty to respect the autonomy of the patient. Consent, express or implied, must be obtained prior to any medical intervention if the patient is a competent adult. If consent is withheld, the doctor is bound by this decision

(*Malette* v. *Schulman*, 1990; *re F*, 1990; *re T*, 1992). If the doctor acts against the wishes of the patient he or she commits a battery, for which he/she may be liable in damages. Obviously, this does not apply if the patient is incapable of consenting.

Elderly patients form a very heterogeneous population. At one end of the spectrum, there are those who are mentally and physically fit apart from the one problem for which they seek medical advice. Such patients may be able to articulate their needs clearly and may be well aware of the nature of the treatment they seek. They may ask about the side-effects of therapy and make it clear to their doctor that they wish to be left with the decision about whether to accept or reject investigation or treatment. At the other end of the spectrum, there are those who are frail with multiple medical problems. They may be able to communicate their needs only poorly, have little understanding of their medical problems and scant knowledge of the help available.

It is tempting, but ethically wrong, for the doctor to assume that these frail patients have a lesser degree of autonomy. It is easy to infantilize patients who cannot easily communicate their needs. Although, in many instances, the patient may be quite happy to leave the decision making to the doctor, this fact should never be assumed. All patients have the right to be consulted about whether they wish to take part in making decisions about their medical care. All capable adult patients must give consent before any form of care or therapy is started. But who is capable and who is not?

CAPACITY AND INCAPACITY

Capacity is a legal concept. However, in practice, assessment of capacity is best done by the doctor caring for the patient. Legally, everyone is presumed to have the mental capacity to make decisions until the contrary is proven. It is the responsibility of the doctor undertaking any particular therapy to judge whether the patient has the capacity to give consent. A patient who lacks the capacity for one decision may be capable of consenting or withholding consent for another. Moreover, patients with fluctuating mental states may be capable of making a decision at one time but not at another. Thus, a judgement of capacity is particular to the decision being made and to the time of the assessment.

Capacity
- Needs to be judged
- Is present until proven otherwise
- May vary by decision and with time

Judging capacity

Capacity for making decisions can be judged using this checklist of five items (BMA/Law Society, 1995).

- The patient should be able to understand in simple language what the medical treatment is, its purpose and nature, and why the treatment is being proposed.
- The patient should understand its principal benefits, risks and alternatives.
- The patient should understand in broad terms the consequences of not receiving the proposed treatment.
- The patient should possess the capacity to make a free choice (free from pressure).
- The patient should retain the information long enough to make an effective decision.

Enhancing capacity by empowering the individual

Many frail elderly patients have multiple problems which impede their capacity to make decisions. Illness affecting speech, hearing, sight, language function, memory, and other cognitive functions are very common in the elderly. All too often such patients are assumed to be incapable of making their own decisions. **The aim should be to empower the patient.** Decisions should not be taken for competent patients unless they have given permission. Discussion with a relative is not a substitute for discussion with a patient if he/she has the capacity to make decisions for him/herself. In cases of borderline capacity doctors should explore means by which communication can be improved and capacity enhanced. Many patients present with highly individual problems demanding unique solutions. It should be possible to devise simple methods to promote autonomy, even in a busy health system.

The three following care illustrations show what can happen when autonomy is ignored, and provide simple ways to enhance capacity (Case studies 2.1–2.3).

Case study 2.1

An elderly Indian woman was admitted to hospital. She could not speak English. In general many decisions were made about investigations without her consent. The discussions about investigation and treatment were often with a family member who could speak English. An independent translator was not used. The family members were rarely used as translators per se, but simply allowed to pass on such information as they felt appropriate. As a result, there was no clear knowledge of whether the patient understood the nature of the investigations and the diagnosis. Her autonomy had been ignored.

Case study 2.2
A 75-year-old female patient with dementia and dysphasia following a stroke was reviewed at the Day Hospital for investigation of diarrhoea. It was initially felt that she had little understanding of her problems and she was treated in her best interests. Little effort was made to find out what she wanted. It was noted that she was deaf. Correction of this problem by way of a hearing aid made some improvements, but communication remained difficult.

She was much less anxious, and communication was improved, when she was not with her daughter. She was interviewed by a sympathetic nurse who established a good rapport with her and, as a result, it became clear that she did not wish further investigation of her diarrhoea and merely wanted symptomatic treatment.

Case study 2.3
An independent elderly woman developed bilateral carpal tunnel syndrome. She was advised that operative intervention was appropriate. Although she trusted the physiotherapists she had little faith in surgical techniques and initially refused an operation. A meeting was arranged between her and another patient who had undergone such surgery. Following this she became more receptive to the idea of operative intervention and underwent decompressive surgery.

Enhancing autonomy

Practical steps can be taken to enhance autonomy.

1. Identify and correct, if possible, handicaps resulting from:
   (i) disease involving hearing, speech, language
   (ii) disease affecting eyesight
   (iii) anxiety and depression
   (iv) memory dysfunction.
2. Allow patients time for decision making.
3. Give adequate information to allow decision making.
4. If necessary, explain the concepts and the decisions more than once.
5. If necessary, write the problems down for the patient.
6. Encourage discussion with relatives or friends.
7. If appropriate, use translators, ideally not always family members.

> **Quality example**
> Steps to enhance autonomy

Planning ahead

In many instances patients can be encouraged to plan ahead. Decisions about various care options are better made if the patient is already familiar with the available choices. Fit elderly patients can be made aware of local residential and nursing homes and of the range of available domiciliary services should they become unable to look after themselves.

The following checklist can be used to compile the relevant information to help the fit elderly with their forward planning.

1. Local nursing and residential homes.
2. Addresses of Age Concern and other charities.
3. Available local social services and addresses of neighbourhood offices.
4. Information on benefits and allowances.
5. Information on home aids and appliances.
6. Information on local day centres and hospitals.
7. Information on common conditions affecting mobility, memory and continence.

Quality example
Forward planning checklists

ADVANCE DIRECTIVES

The purpose of advance directives (or living wills) is to carry autonomy forward to periods of incapacity. Without an advance directive, those patients who do not possess the capacity to give or withhold consent for a particular therapy can be treated under English Law in their 'best interests' (*re F*, 1990; *Airedale NHS Trust* v. *Bland*, 1993).

Under English law a relative or next of kin does not have the legal authority to consent for another adult. It is the doctor who is left with the often difficult task of deciding what is in the patient's 'best interests'.

Without capacity decision are:
• made by doctors
• in patients' best interests
• cannot be made by relatives

One of the problems with 'best interests' is that it has not been clearly defined. As a result of this the Law Commission, in its report on mental incapacity, recommended that in deciding what is in a person's best interest regard should be had to:

(1) the ascertainable past and present wishes and feelings of the person concerned, and the factors that person would consider if able to do so;
(2) the need to permit and encourage the person to participate, or to improve his or her ability to participate,

as fully as possible in anything done for and any decision affecting him or her;

(3) the views of other people whom it is appropriate and practicable to consult about the person's wishes and feelings and what would be in his or her best interests;

(4) whether the purpose for which any action or decision is required can be as effectively achieved in a manner less restrictive of the person's freedom of action. (Law Commission, 1995)

Since the mid-1970s, legislation has been developed in the USA permitting the use of advance statements (living wills) and proxies, whereby a competent person can make anticipatory decisions about future medical care or can nominate another to take such decisions on his or her behalf (Kennedy and Grubb, 1994).

The issue of patient autonomy was forcefully brought to the attention of the American public by the Cruzan case of 1990. Nancy Cruzan had been left in a persistent vegetative state after a car crash in 1983. Although she had not drafted a living will, she had previously indicated informally that if she were permanently unconscious she would not want to be kept alive indefinitely on a life-support machine. The US Supreme Court indicated that, although the constitutional right to refuse treatment survives the loss of decision making capacity, individual states may erect very strict standards of evidence of the incompetent adults former wishes (*Cruzan* v. *Director, Missouri Department of Health*, 1990; Pearlman *et al.*, 1991; Arras. 1991).

In the wake of this case, the US Federal Government passed the Patient Self-Determination Act, 1990 which, *inter alia*, requires hospitals, nursing homes and hospices receiving federal funds to advise patients at the time of admission of their right to make an advance statement.

The act has been criticized because the point of admission may, in many cases, be too late or too insensitive a time to make patients aware of their rights in respect of advance directives (La Puma *et al.*, 1991). It does, however, reflect a move in the USA towards increasing patient autonomy during periods of incapacity. Various other countries have also passed statutes giving effect to advance directives or proxies. The importance of patient autonomy is rapidly becoming a global issue.

US experience
- Case law – the Cruzan case
- Legislation – Patient Self-Determination Act, 1990

UK position
- Case law suggests advance directives may be binding
- No legislation

Quality example
How to judge a living will

Alternatives to living wills
- Durable power of attorney (USA)
- Tutor dative (Scotland)
- None in rest of UK – possible role for informal recording of wishes

In the UK there is currently no legislation governing the use of advance directives or proxies. Recent common law cases have, however, made it increasingly clear that an advance statement indicating a refusal of therapy will bind the doctor provided certain conditions are fulfilled (*re T*, 1992; *Airedale NHS Trust* v. *Bland*, 1993).

Although a patient can authorize or refuse treatment by way of a statement, the patient cannot force the doctor to provide a specific therapy.

Criteria indicating that an advance statement is binding would be that the person:

- was competent when the statement was signed;
- had contemplated the situation which had since arisen;
- appreciated the consequences of refusing treatment;
- was not unduly influenced by another.

Although a legally binding advance statement goes some way towards extending the autonomy of the patient, it cannot cover all the circumstances and decisions that have to be made for an incapacitated patient; it thus remains a useful but blunt instrument. In the USA, an attorney under a durable power of attorney is entitled to make decisions in respect of the medical treatment of incapacitated patients. Although in Scotland a tutor dative can make such decisions, in England, Wales and Northern Ireland these decisions rest solely with the doctor who must act in the patient's 'best interests'. Both the Law Commission and the Scottish Law Commission recommend UK legislation which would enable a mentally competent adult to nominate an attorney who would be capable of taking health care decisions on his/her behalf should he/she become mentally incapable (Law Commission, 1995; Scottish Law Commission, 1995). Both Commissions are also in favour of clarifying the law on advance statements and setting it on a statutory footing.

As a further aid to maintaining autonomy, it might be helpful for patients to document their wishes about future care in a more general and less legalistic way than a legally binding advance statement would allow. It is foreseeable that such an informal record of patients' wishes could be made and kept by general practitioners, and made available to the treating doctors in the event of patients becoming incapacitated. Indeed, although not formal enough to be considered legally binding, any known general expression of wishes by a patient should carry substantial ethical weight in the determination of that patient's 'best interests'.

A series of open questions such as those suggested below may enhance dialogue during informal recording of a patient's wishes.

1. How do you feel about hospitals and hospital investigations?
2. How do you see your future?
3. How would you like to be treated should you become seriously ill?
4. Is it important to you to die in your own home?
5. Is there a member of your family or a friend whom you would like to assist doctors making decisions about your care if you become unable to make such decisions yourself?

EUTHANASIA

Euthanasia continues to be an area of debate internationally.

USA

In the USA, controversy surrounds Dr Jack Kevorkian who in 1996 was, for the second time, acquitted of charges that he illegally assisted in the suicide of two ill patients (Roberts, 1996). In November 1994, voters in Oregan approved Measure 16, permitting physician assisted suicide. Its implementation was, however, blocked by a federal judge, on the day that it was due to become law, on the basis that it was unconstitutional (Charatan, 1994). Although a federal appeals court has, more recently, ruled that mentally competent terminally ill patients have the right to a doctor's assistance in hastening their deaths, the American Medical Association remains of the opinion that physician assisted suicide is unethical and contrary to the role of physician as healer (Macready, 1996).

The Netherlands

At the end of 1993 the Dutch senate passed legislation confirming that euthanasia remained a criminal offence, but formalizing the voluntary procedure by which doctors report euthanasia to the coroner. In practice, doctors following the guidelines set down by the Royal Dutch Medical Association (KNMG) are virtually guaranteed from prosecution (Sheldon, 1993; Scheper *et al.*, 1994). The KNMG guidelines were most recently updated in 1995.

Canada

Although euthanasia remains illegal in Canada, a survey by the Canadian Medical Association and the Toronto Centre for Bioethics in June 1992 showed that 35% of doctors favoured some modification in the criminal code to permit euthanasia (Spurgeon, 1993).

Australia

Australia's first voluntary euthanasia bill became law on 1 July 1996. The Act, which allows doctors in the Northern Territory to assist mentally competent adults who are terminally ill and suffering severe pain to end their lives, has been the subject of much controversy (Zinn, 1996). As in the case of the American Medical Association, the Australian Medical Association opposes physician assisted suicide and euthanasia.

UK

The British Medial Association takes the view that euthanasia is unethical. In 1994, the UK government endorsed the House of Lords Select Committee's rejection of the case for legalizing euthanasia (Government Response to the Report of the Select Committe on Medical Ethics, 1994).

Elderly people form a vulnerable groups. Some may feel pressurized into considering euthanasia simply to avoid becoming a burden to their carers. It is more important that their worries are directly addressed by developing an adequate system of social and palliative care.

RATIONING AND JUSTICE

In the UK, the National Health Service (NHS) was established to right the wrongs of an inequitable system of health care. During the 1930s, medical services were spread unevenly and a large number of poor people were not covered by the national insurance scheme. The new system aimed to provide an equitable service according to need, irrespective of wealth or geographical location.

Although it was initially envisaged that the service would be comprehensive and free at the point of delivery, it became increasingly clear that this was politically unattainable. Prescription charges were introduced in 1951 and thereafter charges for dental and ophthalmic treatment. The most radical and dramatic assault on the original principles has been the shedding by the NHS of its responsibility for continuing care, made possible by a change to social security regulations in 1980.

More recent legislation separating purchaser from provider has highlighted rationing as a major issue within the NHS. Indeed, most would agree that rationing exists in all health care systems. In the past, rationing in the NHS was mostly implicit and based more on traditional modes of practice than on any logical reasoning. This led to decisions that were unjust and unethical. There are several possible bases for rationing.

> **Options for rationing**
> • Age
> • Desert
> • Need
> • Utility

Rationing by age

Health care has been extensively rationed and in some circumstances continues to be rationed on the basis of age. In the past it was assumed that the needs of the elderly were less important than those of the young, and that the elderly would benefit less from treatment. Such assumptions did not take the heterogeneous nature of the elderly population into account, and were based on little scientific evidence.

Although there is now a widespread recognition that many elderly patients respond well to specialist acute care, there are still areas of discrimination: in the UK, unlike in Germany, France and Italy, elderly people are rarely considered for renal replacement therapy (Wing, 1983); there has been a bias against cardiological interventions in the elderly (Elder *et al.*, 1991; Dudley *et al.*, 1992; Topol *et al.*, 1992; Hannaford *et al.*, 1994); elderly patients with cancer are too often referred for palliative care instead of curative treatment (Samet *et al.*, 1986; Greenfield *et al.*, 1987; Fentiman *et al.*, 1990). And yet there is increasing evidence that, if carefully selected, elderly patients benefit substantially from interventions to which they have previously been denied access (Taube *et al.*, 1983; Winearls *et al.*, 1992; Neves *et al.*, 1994). Furthermore, the accurate diagnosis and appropriate treatment of acute illness in elderly patients improves outcome and reduces the inappropriate use of long-stay resources. There can be no doubt that rationing on the basis of age alone is unjust.

> **Examples of ageism**
> • Renal replacement
> • Cardiac care
> • Cancer care

Rationing by desert

Some assert that the treatment of patients who have contributed to their illness through their lifestyle should be of lesser priority – referred to as rationing by desert (Chadwick, 1993). Although the concept may have a 'gut instinct' appeal, as a method of rationing it is ethically flawed. It is not within the role of doctors to 'punish' those who have contributed to their ill health. It is not ethical to abandon people on the grounds of disapproval of their lifestyle.

Rationing according to need

Allocating funds according to need has been seen as an equitable form of rationing in the NHS for many years. From 1976 to 1990, a national formula elaborated by the Resource Allocation Working Party (RAWP) was used to allocate budgets to the regional health authorities. The formula, initially based on age-standardized bed use and then by standardized mortality ratios, was intended to be a convenient proxy for need. In 1990 the formula was again changed to one based on all cause standardized mortality ratio for those aged under 75 years.

Most regions adopted a similar approach for distributing funds to districts. Although this system of weighted capitation has recently been described by the OECD (Organization for Economic Co-operation and Development) as 'one of the most sophisticated and effective means of allocating health resources to areas of need' (OECD Economic Survey UK, 1994), it has also been criticized (Judge et al., 1994).

Further revision takes less account of age and more of socioeconomic factors (Smith et al., 1994). This system has not applied to primary and social care, both of which have been funded by different mechanisms.

It is important that the funding of hospital services, community medical services and community social care is by way of an integrated system. A fragmented system will inevitably lead to the inappropriate use of resources simply to reduce the costs to one particular budget, irrespective of the cost consequences to other budgets. The distribution of such funds to all services should be by way of an equitable system based on the needs of the local population. Rationing according to need would appear to be a system well suited to the allocation of funds to purchasers. However, providers must also take into account the benefits and costs of interventions in addition to a measure of perceived need when allocating funds.

Rationing according to utility

Utilitarianism is a philosophy associated with maximizing benefit. According to the utility model, the aim of rationing should be to maximize the outcome of care. There is, however, a lack of data available on outcomes and cost, and a lack of agreement on how both should be measured. Only 10% to 20% of medical practices are backed up by well designed, randomized controlled trials (Eddy *et al.*, 1992). The analysis of costs within the NHS is similarly at a primitive state of development. The present lack of such data hinders effective rationing on this basis.

Outcome measures have traditionally been used as a method of comparing medical interventions in research. More recently they have started to be used for clinical audit and, more controversially, for comparing the performance of clinical units. Ethically sound rationing on the basis of clinical benefit will depend upon the careful and appropriate use of such data. The UK Clearing House for Information on the Assessment of Health Services Outcomes has recently stared an advisory service on outcome measures (Long *et al.*, 1993).

Outcome measures can be broadly divided into professional measures and patient-centred measures. Professional measures include such examples as mortality statistics, bed occupancy figures, readmission rates and the incidence of specific side-effects. These are often easy to measure and are of undoubted value, but by themselves they cannot be regarded as adequate measures of outcome in elderly patients.

The assessments of disability and handicap are probably the most important outcome measures for the chronic diseases so prevalent in the elderly (Harwood, 1994). Disability or activities of daily living (ADL) scales have been used on elderly people for some time. Although some of the scales are validated for particular situations, no single scale can provide a valid measure for all medical interventions. For example, the Barthel (ADL) Index lacks sensitivity to change in its upper and lower ranges. Thus, it is sensitive to change in a rehabilitation ward for elderly patients (Stone *et al.*, 1994), but not in a geriatric day hospital (Parker *et al.*, 1994). The Frenchay Activities Index scores participation in activities such as domestic chores, household maintenance and paid

---

The range of outcome measures
- 'Professional' or service measures
- 'Patient' measures
  - Impairment
  - Disability (activities of daily living – ADL – scale)
  - Handicap
  - Satisfaction

employment and is thus affected by age, sex and social and cultural status, and the Nottingham Extended ADL scale has been used in stroke patients but is poorly validated in other populations (Rodgers *et al.*, 1993). New outcome scales, such as the London Handicap scale, are being developed to find a valid outcome measure for general use in elderly care.

With the move away from paternalism in medicine, there has been an increasing interest in patient and carer satisfaction as an outcome measure. The validity of many patient satisfaction questionnaires has not been tested. Most patients seem to express high levels of overall satisfaction, which brings into question the sensitivity of the surveys (Whitfield *et al.*, 1992).

However, surprisingly high levels of dissatisfaction can also be found. A recent study revealed that 54% of people with stroke felt they had not had enough therapy (physiotherapy, speech therapy and occupational therapy) (Pound *et al.*, 1994).

Furthermore, carers and patients may have different priorities and views on satisfaction (Jones *et al.*, 1994).

Any system of rationing on the basis of utility will only be successful if information on outcome and cost is readily available to clinicians and managers. The international Cochrane Collaboration was set up to evaluate the evidence available on outcomes from randomized controlled trials. Its goal, to complete a register of all completed and continuing randomized controlled trials and systematic reviews, will, in theory, assist practitioners in rationing care on the basis of outcome. However, the Cochrane Collaboration has been criticized for placing too little emphasis on disseminating the results of its reviews (Godlee, 1994).

Assembling the evidence – the international Cochrane Collaboration.

The increasing availability of CD-ROM and on-line computer links will make the communication of such data considerably easier, but all professionals will have to become familiar with contemporary informatics systems to provide high quality care.

Other approaches to rationing

Despite the lack of data available on outcomes, there is an increasing need for an overt and just system of rationing health care, both in the UK and worldwide. In February 1994, the US state of Oregon began its programme to provide every person in the state with medical and dental services. Like every other state in the USA, Oregon had previously

Other possibilities
• The Oregon experiment
• Core therapy concept

provided Medicaid to only the poorest of its citizens. Although this resulted in 257 000 people qualifying for a comprehensive system of care, it left about 120 000 Oregonians below the poverty line uncovered, and a further 360 000 above the poverty line unable to get insurance.

The new system was set up to ration services and not people. A Health Services Commission, comprising professionals and lay people, heard evidence from both doctors and public groups and drew up a list of 565 conditions to be provided by the state service. The new system has had an enthusiastic response but the implications for cost are as yet uncertain (Roberts, 1994).

In 1992, the Dunning Commission in The Netherlands similarly recommended, as a method of rationing, a core of therapies to which all have equal access. Necessary, effective and efficient care that could not be left to individual responsibility was to be included in the core (Scheerder, 1993). The major problem with the Dunning approach is deciding which particular forms of care should be included in the core.

Future directions in rationing

The Oregon experience is a drastic response to a system of care that is perceived by many as being highly inequitable. In the UK, the NHS already embodies the principle of free access by all citizens to medical care. However, doctors and managers within the NHS are being encouraged to develop explicit policies on prioritization despite the lack of data on outcome and cost. But who should make rationing decisions and how should such decisions be made when there is scant information on outcomes and cost?

The role of purchasers

Rationing decisions should not be left entirely within the hands of purchasers, but there is already evidence that this is occuring. A better role for purchasers would be to encourage providers to analyse and ration the care they provide according to validated outcome measures and cost. Furthermore, it is easy to forget the public in the preset preoccupation with purchasers and providers. The public had an important role in the Oregon experience and it is surely right that they have a role to play in the rationing debate in the UK. The mechanism by which they can be included in such decisions is, however, by no means clear.

Marginal analysis, a system involving the gradual movement of funds from interventions of little benefit to interventions of maximum benefit, is an effective method of rationing at a provider level (Cohen, 1994). UK planning guidance for 1995–6 included the object that the NHS should 'invest an increasing proportion of resources in interventions known to be effective and where outcomes can be systematically monitored, and reduce investment in interventions shown to be less effective' (NHS Executive, 1994). Clinical audit provides a valuable mechanism for ensuring that resources are directed to those interventions known to produce the best outcomes.

The role of doctors

The BMA believes that a doctor's ethical duty goes beyond the individual patient to society as a whole (British Medical Association's Ethics, Science and Information Division, 1993). Thus, it is the duty of all doctors to contribute to a system of rationing. Although purchasers have duties to their population, it is the treating doctor who is best able to assess the situation of individual patients. Doctors must take active steps to make explicit the principles that they use in rationing care and to ensure that such principles are ethically sound. Open dialogue between purchasers, providers and the public is essential to the development of such policies (Hayward, 1994).

CONCLUSION

There is mounting concern that health care is becoming increasingly financially driven with little regard for the needs of individual patients. Fundamental to protection of autonomy is the concept of a partnership between the patient and the health care team. Similarly, a just system of rationing will only be realised by way of a partnership between the public and health care professionals.

REFERENCES

Airedale NHS Trust v. *Bland* (1993) 1 All ER 821.

Arras, J. (1991) Beyond Cruzan: individual rights, family autonomy and the persistent vegetative state. *Journal of the American Geriatric Society*, **39**, 1018–24.

British Medical Association's Ethics, Science and Information Division (1993) *Medical Ethics Today: its practice and philosophy*, BMJ Publishing Group, London.

BMA/Law Society (1995) Assessment of Mental Capacity: guidance for doctors and lawyers. British Medical Association, London.

Chadwick, R. (1993) Justice in priority setting, in *Rationing in Action*, British Medical Journal Publication Group, London, pp. 85–95.

Charatan F. (1994) Judge blocks Oregan's assisted suicide measure. *British Medical Journal*, **309**, 1603.

Cohen, D. (1994) Marginal analysis in practice: an alternative to needs assessment for contracting health care. *British Medical Journal*, **309**, 781–4.

Cruzan v. *Director, Missouri Department of Health* (1990) 110 S Ct 2841 (US Sup. Ct).

Dudley, M.J. *et al.* (1992) The influence of age on policies for admission and thrombolysis in coronary care units in the United Kingdom. *Age and Ageing*, **21**, 95–8.

Eddy, D. *et al.* (1992) Medicine, money and mathematics. *ACS Bulletin*, **77**(6), 36–49.

Elder, A.T. *et al.* (1991) Elderly and younger patients selected to undergo coronary angiography. *British Medical Journal*, **303**, 950–3.

re F (a mental patient: sterilization) (1990) 2 AC 1, 2 All ER 545 (HL).

Fentiman, I.S. *et al.* (1990) Cancer in the elderly: why so badly treated? *Lancet*, **355**, 1020–2.

Godlee, F. (1994) The Cochrane Collaboration. *British Medical Journal*, **309**, 969–70.

Government Response to the Report of the Select Committee on Medical Ethics (1994) Cm 2553, HMSO, London.

Greenfield, S. *et al.* (1987) Patterns of care related to age of breast cancer patients. *Journal of the American Medical Association*, **257**, 2766–70.

Hannaford, P. *et al.* (1994) Ageism as explanation for sexism in provision of thrombolysis. *British Medical Journal*, **309**, 573.

Harwood, R. *et al.* (1994) Measuring Handicap, the London handicap scale, a new outcome measure for chronic disease. *Quality in Health*, **3**, 11–16.

Hayward, J. (1994) Purchasing clinically effective care. *British Medical Journal*, **309**, 823–4.

Jones, D. *et al.* (1994) Hospital care and discharge: patients' and carers' opinions. *Age and Ageing*, **23**, 91–6.

Judge, K. *et al.* (1994) A new approach to weighted capitation. *British Medical Journal*, **309**, 1031–2.

Kennedy, I. and Grubb, A. (1994) Medical Law: Text with Materials, 2nd edn, Butterworths, London, p. 1334.

La Puma, J. *et al.* (1991) Advance directives on admission, clinical implications and analysis of the Patient Self-Determination Act of 1990. *Journal of the American Medical Association*, **266**(3), 402–5.

Law Commission (1995) Mental Incapacity Law Com No 231. London: HMSO.

Long, A.F. *et al.* (1993) The outcomes agenda: contribution of the UK clearing house on health care outcomes. *Quality in Health Care*, **2**, 49–52.

Macready, N. (1996) Assisted suicide is legal, says US judge. *British Medical Journal*, **312**, 655.

Malette v. *Schulman* (1990) 67 (4th) 321 (Ont CA).

Neves, P. *et al.* (1994) Chronic haemodialysis for very old patients. *Age and Ageing*, **23**, 356–9.

NHS Executive (1994) *NHS Executive Priorities and Planning Guidance for the NHS 1995/6*, El 94 55, NHS Executive, Leeds.

OECD Economic Survey UK (1994).

Parker, S.G. *et al.* (1994) Measuring outcomes in care of the elderly. *Journal of the Royal College of Physicians*, **28**, 428–33.

Pearlman, R. *et al.* (1991) Clinical fallout from the Supreme Court decision of Nancy Cruzan: Chernobyl or Three Mile Island? *Journal of the American Geriatric Society*, **39**, 92–7.

Pound, P. *et al.* (1994) Patients' satisfaction with stroke services. *Clinical Rehabilitation*, **8**, 7–17.

Roberts, J. (1996) Kevorkian cleared again. *British Medical Journal*, **312**, 656.

Rodgers, H. *et al.* (1993) Standardised functional assessment scales for elderly patients. *Age and Ageing*, **22**, 161–3.

Samet, J. *et al.* (1986) Choice of cancer therapy varies with age of patient. *Journal of the American Medical Association*, **255**, 3385–90.

Scheerder, R. (1993) Dutch choices in health care, in *Rationing in Action*, British Medical Journal Publishing Group, London, pp. 49–58.

Scheper, T. *et al.* (1994) Euthanasia: the Dutch experience. *Age and Ageing*, **23**, 3–8.

Scottish Law Commission (1995) Report on Incapable adults. Scotland: HMSO.

Sheldon, T. (1993) Euthanasia law does not end debate in The Netherlands. *British Medical Journal*, **307**, 1511.

Smith, P. *et al.* (1994) Allocating resources to health authorities; result and policy implications of small area analysis of use of inpatient services. *British Medical Journal*, **309**, 1050–4.

Spurgeon, D. (1993) Canadian doctors want advice on euthanasia. *British Medical Journal*, **307**, 1378.

Stone, S. *et al.* (1994) The Barthel index in clinical practice: use on a rehabilitation ward for elderly people. *Journal of the Royal College of Physicians of London*, **28**, 419–23.

re T (adult: refusal of treatment) (1992) 4 All ER 649.

Taube, D. *et al.* (1983) Successful treatment of middle aged and elderly patients with end stage renal disease. *British Medical Journal*, **286**, 2018–20.

Topol, E.J. *et al.* (1992) Thrombolytic therapy for elderly patients. *New England Journal of Medicine*, **327**, 45–7.

Whitfield, M. *et al.* (1992) Measuring patient satisfaction for audit in general practice. *Quality in Health Care*, **1**, 151–2.

Winearls, C.G. *et al.* (1992) Age and dialysis. *Lancet*, 339, 432.

Wing, A.J. (1983) Why don't the British treat more patients with kidney failure? *British Medical Journal*, **287**, 1157–8.

Zinn, C. (1996) Australia's doctors battle over euthanasia. *British Medical Journal*, **312**, 1437.

Recent health system developments 3

Gillian B. Todd

EDITORS' INTRODUCTION

Having examined the perspectives of consumers in the last two chapters, we now turn to the second main influence on the quality of care. This chapter gives a comprehensive description of the effects of changes in policy and law on the health care of elderly people, using case studies. The key environmental influence on the quality of care comes from the activities of central government in controlling and changing services through reorganizations.

This chapter comprises two main parts, organized in seven sections. First there is a brief history of the reorganization of the NHS, emphasizing the various motives for the many reorganizations the NHS has experienced. This is expanded upon by examining why and how services for elderly people have changed.

The second part looks in much greater detail at four major changes – commissioning, trusts, GP fundholding, and the Community Care Act, 1990. This explains what commissioners are trying to do and how agencies can work together in needs assessment. The role of trusts is discussed in relation to the development of local policy through teamwork and partnership. GP fundholding is a highly controversial area which Dr Todd attempts to demystify by comparing the utopian vision with the practical tensions that need to be solved. Finally, getting the Community Care Act, 1990 to work constructively is illustrated with a further case study on social workers in primary health care teams.

In this chapter readers will find almost all they need to know about how the map of care has been changed and reorganized. Although many who work in a changing system

Key topics
- History of reorganization
- Elderly people's services
- Commissioning
- Trust creation
- GP fundholding
- The NHS and Community Care Act, 1990

Quality Care for Elderly People. Edited by Peter P. Mayer, Edward J. Dickinson and Martin Sandler. Published in 1997 by Chapman & Hall, London. ISBN 0 412 61830 3

will feel demoralized and disorientated, this chapter offers a positive approach that should revitalize development efforts. There are clear links between the rise of consumerism and some policy changes that focus on basing services on need. This chapter makes a bridge to those that follow: for example, some quality issues are introduced, which are expanded upon in Chapter 4. Importantly, the discussion of relationships and joint working headlines much of what is discussed in Part Two and Part Three.

HISTORY OF REORGANIZATION

Why reorganize?
- For a better balance between hospital and community care
- For a better balance between acute and chronic care
- For greater efficiency
- For higher quality

The National Health Service (NHS) has undergone four major organizational changes in the past 20 years with 1996 seeing a coming together of Family Health Service Authorities and District Health Authorities to form commissioning authorities known as Health authorities. The opportunity was taken to ensure the new authorities are co-terminus with one or more unitary or local authority.

Writing about the 1974 reorganization, the Office of Health Economics reported:

> Although the 1946 Act establishing the NHS represented a skilled and workable compromise between the interests and beliefs of the various groups involved in health care planning and delivery at that time, developments over the past 25 years have made a structural reorganization increasingly necessary. The dominance of hospital-based attitudes and values throughout the NHS and poor liaison between staff working in the community services and those in the hospitals have led to imbalances of care. The problems of the handicapped and the chronically ill in particular have received unsatisfactory attention.

The publication also goes on to point out that between 1946 and 1974 the NHS was also affected by a large number of other factors, such as the Mental Health Act, 1959, the 1966 revision in the contract terms of general practitioners (GPs) and the cogwheel reports.

Since that time the NHS has similarly been regularly influenced by reports, Acts of Parliament, and the results of enquiries. The subsequent reorganizations in 1982, 1984 and 1991 were motivated by the desire to improve the delivery of the service, decrease the administrative costs, and ensure that those responsible for direct patient care have a greater influence on how the service is provided.

In addition, there have been changes in the pattern of resource allocation and in professional training, which have challenged all who work within the service. Throughout this time the service has remained free at the point of delivery, GPs have maintained their independent contractor status, and an improvement in the health of the population and the delivery of high quality service have continued to be the aims of the service. However, there is still concern about imbalances between primary and secondary care, as there was in 1974, and this has resulted in the recent proposals to introduce GP-led purchasing.

CHANGES IN SERVICES FOR ELDERLY PEOPLE

Services for elderly people have also changed during the past 20 years. Much of that change has been driven by clinical advances and the availability of new drugs and medical technology. However, some of it is the result of the organizational, managerial and professional changes that have occurred in the NHS.

There is no doubt that the pace of organizational change has increased very considerably in the past 10 years, even more so in the past four years, and that in addition it has been associated with changed patient and professional expectations and the introduction of general management. General managers in the service now insist on being able to describe in a quantifiable way the performance of the service and the return, in terms of patient care, obtained for the resources invested. Value for money, productivity, cost-effectiveness, and efficiency are top of the agenda. This results in a very different service from that provided in the 1970s, and has led to concern on the part of patients and professionals that it is finance, not quality, led.

The publication in 1989 of *Caring For People* (DoH, 1989a) heralded change in the community care system and was followed by the NHS and Community Care Act, 1990, which was implemented in 1993. The change can be summarized as moving from a supply-led institutionalized service, which was NHS-led, to a needs-led community-based service, which is local government-led. The resources used by the social security system to fund residential care were transferred in 1993 to local authorities, and, together with the resources they had already committed to the provision of community care services, were meant to provide a unified budget from which residential and non-residential care could be

---

Change drivers
- Clinical advances
- Organizational change
- Management
- Patients' expectations

Principal change
- **From** supply, hospital, NHS focus
- **To** needs, community, local government focus

purchased, dependent on the detailed assessment of individual need. These changes have generally been welcomed and implemented successfully, but problems have arisen about the way in which health care and social care are defined. Those who have health care needs are funded free and those with social care needs are means-tested to establish the financial contribution they will be required to make towards their care.

A recent publication entitled *NHS responsibilities for meeting continuing health care needs* (DoH, 1995) makes the broad definitions clear, but requires local detailed agreements between health and local authorities to be in place. There have been a number of court cases, resulting in the establishment of case law. The majority of elderly people live at home and wish to continue to do so; many local authorities have introduced flexible packages of care to make this possible. The needs of the carer are now being considered by many health and local authorities in order to ensure that even more people can remain at home.

Elderly people are major users of health services and of social services. Much of the health care they receive is provided by the primary health care team and community-based services such as chiropody, hearing and eye services. Health and social services work together to provide as much care as possible for elderly people in their own homes or close to where they live. It is hoped that such care will enable elderly people to remain in their own homes. The objective is to provide co-ordinated care between community-provided health services, social service needs-led provision and the primary health care team. This is referred to as 'seamless care'.

The principles and philosophy underlying the present provision of health and social services are, in the main, those described in the 1989 White Papers *Working for patients* (DoH, 1989a) and *Caring for people – community care in the next decade and beyond* (DoH, 1989b), and included in the subsequent NHS and Community Care Act, 1990. These are: first, the separation of those responsible for purchasing and those responsible for providing, so ensuring explicit service provision, using contracts as the mechanism; second, the move of emphasis from secondary to primary and community care using GP-led purchasing and the provision of needs-led health and social care packages as the mechanism. These principles and their effect on services for elderly people are described in more detail below.

Seamless care
Co-ordinating:
- health
- social services
- primary care

Instruments of change
- Commissioning
- Trusts
- GP fundholding
- NHS and Community Care Act, 1990

The publication of *The health of the nation – a strategy for health in England* (DoH, 1993) in 1993, *Promoting Better Health* (DoH, 1987) in 1987 and *The Patient's Charter* (DoH, 1991) in 1991 were all pieces of the same jigsaw: although these White Papers were the result of the work of different bodies, they all point in the same direction. The legislation passed in 1995 has resulted in the integration of district health authorities (DHAs) and family health service authorities (FHSAs), and the guidance issued in relationship to the need to move towards GP-led purchasing with DHAs in support, is a further piece of that puzzle.

COMMISSIONING

There are several key targets to achieve as the commissioning role continues to be developed by health authorities and local authorities.

* Population knowledge
* Needs assessment
* Purchasing plans which respond to need, demand and local problems
* Seamless care for individuals between primary, secondary and tertiary
* Health care and social care
* The continual evaluation of the clinical effectiveness of various types of care
* A focus on the health of the population.

Health authorities, and previously DHAs and FHSAs have been working hard to achieve these targets since 1990, building on the report of the Committee of Inquiry into the Future Development of the Public Health in England (1988). Sir Donald Acheson chaired the inquiry, established by the Secretary of State for Social Services on 21 January, 1986, which made 39 recommendations. Recommendation 4 has considerable significance for the work of commissioning authorities.

We define the public health responsibilities of district health authorities as follows:

1. To review regularly the health of the population for which they are responsible and to identify problems. To define objectives and set targets to deal with the problems in the light of national and regional guidelines.

> **Practice point**
> Commissioners have six key targets to achieve

2. To relate the decisions which they take about the investment of resources to their impact on the health problems and objectives so identified.
3. To evaluate progress towards their stated objectives.
4. To make arrangements for the surveillance, prevention, treatment and control of communicable disease and infection.
5. To give advice to, and seek co-operation with, other agencies and organizations in their locality to promote health.

We consider that this should be the framework within which decisions on priorities and developments should be based and we recommend that DHAs should be required to commission an annual report from their Director of Public Health on the health of the population. In formulating their views about the report they should consult local authorities, FPCs and other relevant bodies locally.

Needs assessment, knowledge of the population and the search for clinically effective care and treatment was further developed in the White Paper *Working For Patients* (DoH, 1989b). The importance of joint working with local authorities and voluntary organizations is a key objective of *Caring for People – Community Care in the Next Decade and Beyond* (DoH, 1989a). There are many examples of collaboration and joint working. The one described here (Case study 3.1) has been selected because it is known to the author, illustrates the creation of a shared planning data base for all the authorities and voluntary organizations concerned with the provision of care in South Glamorgan, and provides an example of how Recommendation 4 of the Acheson report can be put into practice.

Case Study 3.1   Joint needs assessment South Glamorgan health and social care profile – 1993
The profile was put together by a Project Steering Group comprised of representatives from six sponsoring Authorities: the City of Cardiff Council, South Glamorgan County Council, the Vale of Glamorgan Borough Council, South Glamorgan Family Health Services Authority, South Glamorgan Health Authority and South Glamorgan Intervol (the local Voluntary Services Forum).
It had its origins in a proposal in 1991 by a group of staff from the County Council and the health authorities responding to the availability of data from the 1991 population

census and the recommendation of the NHS and Community Care Act, 1990 that services should be provided following assessments of need. The aim was to produce an area profile of the health of South Glamorgan in order to advise the purchasing function for health and social care and the local strategies for health process, which involved the health authorities, the County Council and the district councils in working together. It was intended to enable the monitoring of change and trends from previous census bases, and to promote collaboration between the statutory bodies in the pursuit of their overall health and social care objectives.

The publication was based on data by local government district wards. The profile included chapters on:

- *The population of South Glamorgan*
- *Indicators of health and social care needs*
- *Environmental and other determinants of health*
- *Lifestyle and need*
- *Health and use of health care services*
- *Need and use of social care services*
- *The potential impact of structural change*
- *Comparison of need, demand and supply.*

It included some challenging data in relation to elderly people. The following inserts are reproduced from the document, for illustrative purposes, with permission from South Glamorgan Health Authority.

Lone pensioners

The 1991 population census data showed marked variations within the county for this variable. Figure 3.1 shows the geographical distribution of the percentage of pensioners living alone. It can be seen that this reflects the distribution of elderly people, rather than the distribution of other social variables; however, it is clear that a significant number of these households will require considerable input from the health and social care community services.

Hospitalization rates

The South Glamorgan hospitalization rate in 1991/92 was estimated to be 209 per 1000 population. Females of childbearing ages and immediately beyond were hospitalized more often than males, otherwise the distribution between the sexes were equal. Emergency hospitalization rates were very similar for males and females, and for both sexes they increased markedly above the age of 65 years. Half of those aged 85 and over were admitted as an emergency in 1991/92.

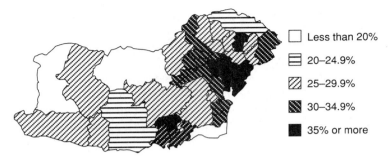

Figure 3.1 Percentage of pensioners living alone in South Glamorgan, by district, 1991. Source: 1991 population census Local Base Statistics, Crown copyright; boundaries copyright of Ordnance Survey.

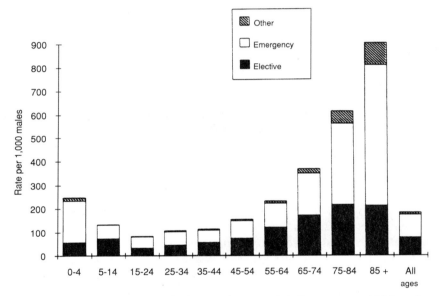

Figure 3.2 Age-specific hospitalization (NHS) rates per 1000 male South Glamorgan residents, 1991/92. Source: based on data from South Glamorgan Health Authority, Mid-Glamorgan Health Services Authority and Glamorgan Health Authority.

Practice point
The need to clarify the planning base:
- localities?
- wards?
- GP lists?

The South Glamorgan Director of Public Health's Annual Report in 1994 contained a chapter entitled 'The Locality Dimension'. It argues for using localities rather than local government district wards, but recognizes the difficulty of

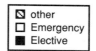

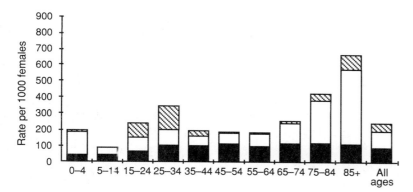

Figure 3.3 Age-specific hospitalization (NHS) rates per 1000 female South Glamorgan residents, 1991/92. Source: based on data from South Glamorgan Health Authority, Mid-Glamorgan Health Services Authority and Glamorgan Health Authority.

creating artificial planning boundaries for health services that are different to those used by other statutory authorities. This debate will become even more vigorous as commissioners work to support GP-led purchasing. The planning and monitoring base for the provision of health care will be the general practice lists, and the Census and Registrar General Data will be local authority ward-based. Many health authorities are tackling this problem and it will be important to share the successes and failures as they occur.

There is a need for a population health and social care profile in each authority area to inform GPs, health authorities, local authorities and others of the problems they need to tackle, and to provide them with a data base as a means of monitoring success.

The result of this should be the:

- targeting of services towards those in greatest need
- identification of unmet need that requires new or different services
- statutory and voluntary organizations working together to provide seamless care
- GPs and the primary health care teams taking responsibility for the health care of the elderly people registered

---

A care profile
- is a shared resource
- informs decisions
- can monitor success

with them and ensuring care is targeted at those most in need.

TRUST CREATION

The fundamental principles underlying the development of trusts are:

- The creation of organizations that are dependent on acquiring income in return for quantified services.
- The involvement of a chairman and non-executive directors in the organization to provide a focus for decision making.

These principles result in trusts producing business plans that describe in detail what they are able to provide, at what quality and at what cost. In the NHS, business plans need the support of commissioning organizations to ensure that trust prices remain appropriate and take account of the full cost of revenue consequences of capital schemes and developments. This control mechanism is of paramount importance – without it a trust would be able to enhance its services, change the range of services, and increase prices without agreement. As a result, commissioning authorities would be unable to continue to purchase the same level of service.

There needs to be a partnership, and both trust and commissioning authority need to agree plans for change. This partnership is important. It should be between two equals: one with expertise in the provision of a high quality service, keen to improve that service in a measured and quantified way, striving for effective care; and the other, keen to agree contracts that provide high quality, cost-effective services targeted at those most in need. A tension should exist in this dialogue and the necessary negotiation, but it should be constructive and result in mutually beneficial change. An example of how such partnerships can exist between commissioners and more than one provider is given in Case Study 3.2.

> The commissioning partnership with a common quality interest.

Case Study 3.2   A policy forum: integration of general medicine and geriatric medicine
The South Glamorgan DHA and FHSA made a decision during 1994 to establish a policy forum in which issues of concern could be debated openly between chairmen, non-executive

members, executive members, provider trusts, GPs, clinicians and nurses. The purpose behind the decision of the commissioners to have such a forum was to ensure that there was an opportunity to discuss complex issues that could involve considerable change, particularly in relation to the pattern of clinical practice, in a relaxed atmosphere, without any pressure to agree a certain way ahead.

In their purchasing intentions in July 1994, the authorities had stated that they wanted to commission general medical and geriatric medical services that were non-discriminatory by age. There was a general awareness of the various models of service provision for general medical and geriatrics that existed within the Trusts the district contracted with as well as those existing in England and Wales. It was felt that the commissioning authority would be unwise to require within contracts an integrated general medical and geriatric medical service without having the opportunity to understand all the issues involved, so a three-part process was undertaken.

A day-long workshop was held to identify the issues that needed to be debated. Speakers were invited to present alternative approaches to the way general medical and geriatric medical services could interface. The workshop involved provider trust managers, clinicians (both geriatricians and general physicians), GPs and members of commissioning teams. The result of the workshop was unexpected: there was a unanimous acceptance of the need to provide an acute medical service that was non-discriminatory by age, in which geriatricians and physicians worked alongside each other in order to ensure that:

- *specialist services were available to all who needed them regardless of age;*
- *those requiring rehabilitation and multidisciplinary care should have access to those services regardless of age;*
- *the acutely ill patient was admitted to an admission unit where nursing skills were high and senior doctors were involved in the care at the onset.*

Consequently, the lively debate that had been expected at the policy forum between physicians and geriatricians, did not take place. Instead, the first workshop suggested that the areas in need of debate were:

- *the relationship between the primary care team and the geriatric service;*

- *the role of community hospitals in the care of the elderly;*
- *the detail of the contract needed for acute medical services.*

The second part of the process was to have a policy forum workshop involving the chairmen, non-executive and executive officers, GPs, trust managers and clinicians. The areas previously identified were addressed, guest speakers introduced the subject, and the following action plan was agreed.

- *An integrated admissions unit, managed by physicians and geriatricians, should be provided in each trust.*
- *Access to specialist services would be according to clinical need, not age.*
- *The configuration of services for elderly people in each locality would be the result of discussion between the GP, the primary health care team, the geriatricians the commissioners, and social services, and would vary depending on the health need and the population size.*
- *An assessment would be made by the commissioner of the opportunities that exist for increasing the size of the primary health care teams in order to enable them to increase the amount of care provided to elderly people.*

The third part of the process was to get the policy direction approved by the DHA and FHSA.

Practice point
With the right setting, people will work together to develop services

---

The significance of this Case Study 3.2 is that it demonstrates partnership, a willingness to recognize that the issues that may have been considered to be the most difficult may in fact not be, and finally that the way forward between trusts and commissioners must be that of a regular dialogue for mutual learning and exploring the issues. In contrast, aggressive contracting, based on misconceptions about the everyday problems of providing care, could lead to a concentration on issues of less importance and a consequent neglect of the areas where changes may be most beneficial.

The trusts and GPs are in an admirable position to be aware of carer and patient satisfaction. The expectation of commissioners is that trusts will be proud of what they achieve and the commissioner will not have to persuade them to measure clinical outcomes or patient satisfaction. The setting up of trusts aimed to ensure that there was a pride at local level in the provision of the service, which should result in making the most of success. Commissioners need to be partners in encouraging this success.

GP FUNDHOLDING

GP fundholding and GP-led purchasing, along with the move in many commissioning authorities towards locality-based planning and commissioning, is an important part of the NHS changes since 1990. There has been much criticism of GP fundholding, but there is no doubt that it has encouraged a number of important changes in thinking about how services should be planned, commissioned and provided. GPs and the primary health care teams have a responsibility to provide a service to an identified group of patients. In the 1970s and 1980s, management teams often had GP representation, but in general the influence of GPs on the services provided was small, and the influence of the consultant body was greater. As we have already seen, the desire in 1974 was to create a health service with more balance between primary and secondary care. The changes made between 1991 and 1995 would appear to provide a greater chance of success. There are, however, many pitfalls and problems to overcome if a true balance is to be attained between primary care and its associated community care and secondary care.

> **GP fundholding**
> • Much criticized
> • A catalyst for change
> • Symbol of primary care emphasis
> • The vision of comprehensive integrated local care.

At its simplest, GP-led purchasing will result in GPs building up their primary health care teams, working in conjunction with social services and neighbouring practices to provide local emergency care centres – specialized outpatient and residential care services – thus minimizing the need for secondary care. Secondary care services will be purchased on a cost per case basis and patients will be referred where the quality and access to care is best. Dissatisfied patients will lead to changes in referral patterns. However, it is not as simple as that.

The NHS has a responsibility and an accountability to ensure that the public money invested in it is used in the best way possible. It has a responsibility to address the health of the population as a whole and to ensure that, for example, infectious diseases are controlled, screening programmes are available to those who fit the criteria, and child protection services are provided. This means that GPs need to take account of wider issues and to purchase within the framework agreed by national initiatives. Health authorities must therefore set up a robust planning mechanism that ensures that GPs are fully aware of the national imperatives and are involved in producing local plans.

> **Tensions**
> • Local v. national
> • Short-term v. long-term
> • Primary v. secondary care

The challenge that health authorities have in working with GPs to achieve this close working relationship from a planning point of view, is that GPs' prime focus is on today's care issues, rather than planning for the future. The development by many authorities of locality planning teams is aimed at achieving this framework in a way that ensures the cooperation of GPs.

Primary health care teams and local social services work primarily with elderly people and the chronically sick. The move to GP-led purchasing, locality-based population needs assessment, and close working relationships between social services, voluntary organizations and the primary health care team has the potential to achieve major changes in the provision of services to elderly people. Such services would be locally sensitive and aimed at providing care in local communities.

The second area of concern is that many secondary care providers may be destabilized as more is invested in primary and community care. This will lead inevitably to a restructuring of the secondary care sector. The secondary care sector faces many difficulties, not least the restructuring of the conditions of junior doctors, and a need to ensure that the care provided to patients has an outcome that is equivalent to the best in the country. High quality effective secondary care is dependent on the availability of intensive and high dependency care, a comprehensive range of diagnostic and other investigatory services and multispecialty specialist expertise. This means that there is an optimum size for a hospital and that it will also need to ensure that it is able to keep pace with national changes in care from a research, development and training point of view. This will be the challenge of the 21st century as expectations rise, outcomes become more important and local communities want local acute services.

THE COMMUNITY CARE ACT, 1990

The implementation of the Community Care Act, 1990 has resulted in a considerable amount of change in the pattern of service to elderly people or those requiring support in daily living activities. There are many examples of very innovative packages of care that enable patients to be cared for in their own homes. The act has necessitated close working relationships between social service departments and health authorities. Case Study 3.3 shows an example of this.

Case Study 3.3   Attachment of social workers to primary health care teams in South Glamorgan
The challenge to primary health care teams, social services and voluntary organizations is to establish firm mechanisms whereby seamless services are available to those in need. One mechanism for doing this is to attach social workers to primary health care teams. A recent evaluation of such a scheme in South Glamorgan was positive, as a result of which both the FHSA and social services decided to extend the initiative.

In 1991, following discussions with social services, the FHSA piloted the attachment of a medical social worker to a primary health care team in Ely, Cardiff. The outcome of the pilot scheme is described below from the viewpoint of the social worker.

Summary of key points: views from the attachment social worker
High levels of daily informal contact with the core primary health care team (including joint visits) were invaluable as a means of developing awareness about respective skills, expertise and patient needs.

The need for effective systems to monitor hospital admissions and related patient needs has been highlighted by the attachment scheme.

Very few instances of confusion or disagreement arose over the role of the attachment worker in relation to case responsibility among health and social services providers.

The attached social worker was welcomed as a full member of the primary health care team, and was able to influence the way in which referrals were identified. This helped to prioritize need and enhanced job satisfaction.

Joint DHA/FHSA/social services agreement
As a result of the pilot scheme, a steering group was set up to look at the possibility of extending the number of attachments of social workers to primary health care teams.

All GP practices in South Glamorgan were contacted, consulted about the practical issues involved, and their accommodation inspected.

As a result of this process, 19 practices were recommended to receive attached social workers, and 10.5 (full-time equivalent) social workers were made available to the scheme.

Specification for the social work attachment
In outline the attached social workers have three main functions:

- *to undertake a hospital discharge function for patients of the practice;*
- *to provide social case work support to those patients of the practice who have social problems as a result of ill health;*
- *to provide a signposting service to the practice for patients who require access to specialist social care resource centres such as elderly mentally infirm (EMI) teams, child protection teams and resource centres for elderly people.*

The roll out of the scheme is in its early days, but the initiative does offer a number of potential opportunities, particularly in Cardiff where the greatest concentration of attachments is taking place.

In particular, the initiative offers the opportunity for social workers to be perhaps the key primary care workers for children with special needs and to work with new unitary authorities to ensure continuation and continued evaluation of the scheme.

CONCLUSION

We have seen how services for elderly people have been fundamentally affected by recent changes in the organization of the NHS. These changes have the potential to ensure locally responsive primary care-based services with clear agreements in place with social services about supporting social care services. However, they require considerable planning on the part of DHAs, FHSAs, and social service departments to ensure the potential is fully realized. The secondary care trusts will need to make sure their services support such local services and are reconfigured to meet the challenge. The provision of seamless care, particularly between social services and the primary health care team, is essential if the objectives of care are to be met, needs-led, and seamlessly provided, at home if possible.

REFERENCES

Committee of Inquiry into the Future Development of the Public Health in England (1988) *Public health in England*, Cm 289, HMSO, London.

Department of Health (1987) *Promoting better health. The Government's programme for improving primary health care*, Cm 249, HMSO, London.

Department of Health (1989a) *Caring for people – community care in the next decade and beyond*, Cm 849, HMSO, London.

Department of Health (1989b) *Working for patients*, Cm 555, HMSO, London.

Department of Health (1991) *The Patient's Charter*, HMSO, London.

Department of Health (1993) *The health of the nation – a strategy for health in England*, Cm 1986, HMSO, London.

Department of Health (1995) *NHS responsibilities for meeting continuing health care needs*, HSG(95)8, NHS Executive, Leeds.

South Glamorgan Health Authority (1993) *South Glamorgan health and social care profile*, South Glamorgan Health Authority, Cardiff.

The quality movement 4

Edward J. Dickinson

EDITORS' INTRODUCTION

This chapter is mainly concerned with strategic aspects of the quality movement, but detailed information is also included to illustrate key points.

The chapter consists of four sections. The first section presents a short history of the quality movement in business and how this has been translated into public services and then into health services. The second section discusses the broad principles of the quality movement in health care – most importantly, the quality cycle. The third section goes on to introduce the quality toolbox, a concept that is used to help us think about the wide variety of quality activities there are now. This is explained with examples of all the quality tools, and suggests that clinical audit may be more useful to organizations than medical audit, an idea echoed in Chapter 8. The fourth section looks to the future and considers some of the key areas where changes might occur during this decade – the strengthening of management, the cross-fertilization of business experience, and a heightened consumer focus. The conclusion restates the key themes that have been explored.

After reading this chapter, you will have an up-to-date appreciation of the theory and practice of quality improvement. This should assist you in understanding all that is discussed in the rest of this book about quality. For example, Chapter 5 provides a practical approach to setting up a quality initiative and Chapter 7 covers a wide range of quality activities in the private sector. If you are interested in reading more about how to put consumerism into action, again, Chapters 5 and 7 have much to offer which can be applied in other sectors and settings. Thus, this chapter should equip you with knowledge and confidence to discuss quality and set about improving quality in the areas that are important in your area of work.

Key topics
- History of quality
- Quality principles
- Present activity
- The quality toolbox
- A look to the future

Quality Care for Elderly People. Edited by Peter P. Mayer, Edward J. Dickinson and Martin Sandler. Published in 1997 by Chapman & Hall, London. ISBN 0 412 61830 3

Relman's paradigm
- Rapid expansion
- Cost containment
- Accountability

The 1980s were the decade of quality in the commercial world and the 1990s seem set to be the decade of quality in public services. The purpose of this chapter is to provide an overview of the development of quality in health services. The broad context for this change are the three 'revolutions' in developing health care systems (Relman, 1988). First, there is the rapid expansion of services, activity and consequent costs exemplified by the USA in the 1960s. Second, there is the resulting concern about the increasing costs of health care (either of governments or third party payers such as insurance companies). Third, there is the realization that the **quality** of care is of greater importance.

This third revolution can be discerned as a common strand in the changes that have occurred in health systems such as the UK's National Health Service (NHS), and is reflected in the prominence of quality considerations in the health services of many countries around the world. These may be driven by diverse factors: cost concerns may be prominent – there is a general view that striving for quality produces a net saving in costs (Bank, 1992); restructuring may be occurring – in the NHS an internal market has been created and this provides a context in which quality can be made more explicit; or there may be a more overt need to compete – quality is now widely regarded as a key competitive weapon in manufacturing and services (Johnson and Scholes, 1993).

A SHORT HISTORY OF QUALITY

This section examines the roots of the quality movement in health services by describing how the modern quality movement started in the world of manufacturing products, with particular reference to the 'quality gurus'. The translation of this experience into the public sector is then discussed, and then the history of the quality movement in health services is considered.

Quality in manufacturing products

Much of our thinking about quality stems from the influence of the so-called 'quality gurus' such as Deming, Juran, Crosby, and Feigenbaum. Initially, there was concern with the quality of manufactured goods as businesses began to realize that quality was a key ingredient of competitive advantage. The origins of this trend can be traced back to the visits of Deming and Juran to Japan in the 1950s to assist with industrial reconstruction following the Second World War.

Although there has been wide diffusion of quality since, there is also the danger of quality being viewed as a panacea or a fad (Lorenz, 1993).

Although details of the approaches of the quality gurus differ quite markedly, there is much commonality in the principles they propose. Nine common points have been discerned (Ghobadian and Speller, 1994), and these are shown in Box 4.1. They emphasize the importance of people and management in achieving high quality. Such concepts have largely been developed in the context of manufacturing operations, but they are increasingly being translated into service operations. This, in turn, has stimulated a context for increasing interest in applying quality concepts to public sector service organizations and, more recently, to the health service.

In considering the evolution of quality in product manufacture, it becomes clear that there are limitations to the approaches of the gurus (Garvin, 1987; Chase and Aquilano, 1989).

Practice point
How the 'gurus' agree:
- process
- people
- management

Box 4.1   Common themes among the quality gurus

- Control the process, not the product
- Remember the human aspect, not just the technical aspect
- Top management is responsible for quality
- Management needs to foster a quality culture
- Training is essential to enhance staff knowledge and attitudes
- Prevention of quality problems is more important than inspection after the event
- Quality is a long-term commitment not an instant cure
- All activities can be looked at for quality improvement
- Quality is an organization-wide activity

- There is a lack of a firm conceptual framework.
- There is no recognized diagnostic method whereby an organization can examine quality to decide what is needed and which aspects of quality matter.
- It is difficult to apply the concepts of quality to specific circumstances in an organization.

However, the 'gap' model of service quality has potential to solve these problems and appears to be gaining ground in acceptance and use (Parasuraman, Zeithaml and Berry, 1985).

Translation of quality into public services

The quality movement began to diffuse into services when it was realized that the approaches of the gurus could be transferred to this sector. This was strengthened by recognition of the importance of putting the customer first. The quality movement began to influence public services during the 1980s, and in the UK this was initially seen in local government services.

This has been ascribed to factors such as the introduction of compulsory competitive tendering, consumerism, and the cross-fertilization of ideas from dealing with the private sector. In addition, government policy and other central activities have promoted quality through quality campaigns, the British Quality Association, the British Standards Institute, the Audit Commission and several research and development bodies.

Quality in health services

Quality in health services has become increasingly prominent in the past five years. As discussed, the quality movement in health services forms the third revolution in Relmans' development paradigm (1988). Resource awareness, system reorganization and awareness of quality competition may all play a part.

Within the NHS, system reorganization has both created an environment that favours the quality movement, and provided new potent forces for a change to the quality perspective.

The importance, power and potential influence of the **consumer** is now being recognized in health care. This is occurring in the context of a general rise of consumerism in society, and is due to specific changes in health services such as the *Patient's Charter* (Department of Health, 1991), and

---

Quality drivers in public services
- Compulsory competitive tendering
- Consumerism
- Commercial influence
- Government policy
- National activities

delegation of purchasing to primary health care practitioners. These are coupled with a gradual untangling of need and demand, respect for satisfaction as a legitimate outcome measure, and a focus on the views of consumers in the design of high quality services.

The **internal market**, with the split between purchasers and providers with contracts for health care between them, has lead to an emphasis on quality, the need for appropriate health systems and awareness of the cost of operations.

Managerially, quality in health care has benefited from cross-fertilization of ideas from commerce. The gradual strengthening of health service management has brought with it a realization of the importance of quality. Although some initiatives might be criticized as 'window dressing', there is hope that more serious activities will take root, especially at the interface with clinical audit.

New forces have been created in the new NHS which are also at work in promoting quality (Figure 4.1, see later). These include clinical audit (Department of Health, 1993a), clinical guidelines (Scottish Office, 1993), and the idea of science-based care (Department of Health, 1993b).

By and large, the health professions have participated energetically in these changes, building on their traditional activities in maintaining standards. Standard setting has always been an important role for them, particularly in relation to training, qualifications and accreditation of specialists. More recently, the setting of explicit standards for routine care has become more common; bodies such as the medical royal colleges and the chartered societies have all been active in producing national standards of care, especially in respect of the health care of elderly people. Many of these are included in a directory entitled *Gold Standards* (Age Concern, 1994).

Early involvement of clinicians
• Training
• Qualifications
• Accreditation of specialists

An additional trend is the activity of governmental bodies, and this has been particularly noticeable in the long-term care of elderly people (Social Services Inspectorate, 1990).

Managers have also participated in quality, but through less structured activities. Total quality management (TQM) has been espoused by some, but in general organizational initiatives appear to be scarcer, despite encouragement from the Institute of Health Service Managers (1989) and the efforts of the King's Fund organization audit programme (Shaw and Brooks, 1991). This may reflect a lack of strategy and managerial experience, and possible cynicism among front line staff in respect of managerial activities. Such mistrust between managerial and health professionals may also be exemplified by the difficulties that have been experienced in translating the findings of clinical audit into organizational development.

There are two final general points about the quality movement in health care. First, the importance of quality is slowly being recognized externally through competitive awards. Hewlett Packard sponsors the Golden Helix awards, and the newspaper *Hospital Doctor* organizes sponsored awards in many aspects of hospital health care.

Second, a vast range of approaches to quality have appeared. This partly reflects the complexity of health care, but also suggests that much of the work that is being done is fragmented. One consequence is that many staff may be uncertain about what is going on and what part they should play in it. Section four of this chapter seeks to demystify the enormous range of quality activities using the idea of the quality toolbox. But first, the broad principles of quality in health care are described.

Practice point
Staff may be uncertain about:
- what is going on
- their role in it

BROAD PRINCIPLES OF QUALITY IN HEALTH CARE

Three important broad principles have emerged that are relevant to development of the quality movement. First, there is increasing clarity about the meaning of high quality care. One of the best *aides-mémoire* for defining high quality care is the phrase 'doing the right things . . . well', derived from the longer definition of Brook and Kosecoff (1988). This bipartite concept implies the need both for quality standards, which define what should be done, and a quality method for ensuring that it is.

Second, there appear to be four major dimensions to quality in health care, although Maxwell (1984) has described more.

Important quality principles
- Quality can be defined
- Four dimensions of quality
- Cyclical approach

- Effectiveness
- Efficiency
- Equity
- Humanity

The third principle, which is now widely accepted, is the cyclical natural of quality activities. This is well exemplified by the audit cycle (Figure 4.1) and underlines the importance of striving for continuous improvement in quality.

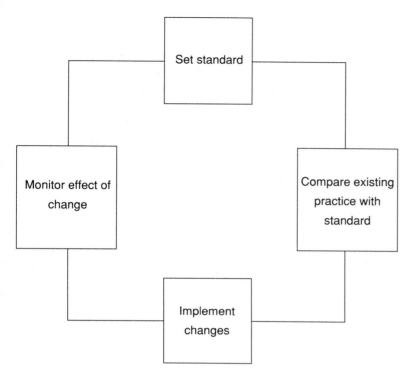

Figure 4.1   The audit cycle.

PRESENT ACTIVITY

This section describes the range of quality activities that are now being carried out, using the concept of the quality toolbox as an explanatory device. The quality toolbox contains four main quality tools – quality methods, quality standards, quality measures and quality support systems. Each tool has a different role but all the tools should be used together for best effect.

- **Quality methods** are the actual schemes of activities that will be carried out by staff, the most common being clinical audit.
- **Quality standards** provide the objectives against which performance is assessed in the quality cycle. These may be derived internally but there is an increasing number of regional and national standards.

Practice Point
The quality toolbox
- Methods – actual activities
- Standards – objectives
- Measures, e.g. outcome measures
- Support systems, e.g. BS 5750

- **Quality measures** are assessments that may be useful in quality assurance, such as outcome and case mix measures.
- **Quality support systems** are the infrastructure to help quality activities work. For example, a new infrastructure, which includes audit staff, has been set up throughout the UK to allow the execution of clinical audit.

Examples of each type of quality tool are discussed below, and a complementary digest of quality initiatives can be found in *A to Z of quality: a guide to quality initiatives in the NHS* (NHS Management Executive, 1993).

Tool 1: quality methods

There has been a proliferation of quality methods. For the purposes of discussion, they can be broadly split into professional and organizational approaches (Box 4.2).

Quality methods
- Professional – clinical audit
- Organizational

Professional

Audit is a required activity, introduced in 1989 (Department of Health, 1989) and now evolving into clinical audit to reflect the patterns of teamwork in routine care (Royal College of Physicians, 1993). Audit has been promoted by the royal colleges as an educational activity (Royal College of Physicians, 1989a, 1993). However, there are major challenges such as time, resources, training and carrying out audit across the care interfaces, which are vital to the quality of care of elderly people. Audit comprises two main types of activities – case note review and topic audit, neither of which is entirely satisfactory. Case note review can easily become repetitive and boring. On the other hand, topic audit can easily mushroom into full-blown research.

A possible way to keep audit meaningful is provided by clinical audit – the theory being that the different disciplines will need to focus on realistic and achievable topic audits in order to make any progress. In retrospect, it seems obvious that audit should have been clinical, rather than medical, from the start, especially in an multiprofessional specialty such as the care of elderly people.

Other quality methods have been developed by other professions. Nurses have been particularly active. The Dynamic Standard Setting System (DySSSy) of the Royal College of Nursing is popular (Royal College of Nursing, 1990). There is also a variety of methods that are particularly concerned with

---

Box 4.2   Quality methods

- Organizational
  Total Quality Management (TQM), Zero Defects, etc.
  Outcomes management
  Critical events monitoring
  Hospital accreditation
- Professional
  Medical audit, clinical audit
  DySSSy
  Qualpacs
  Monitor (various versions)
  CARE scheme
  Quality circles
  National enquiries (e.g. NCEPOD, Maternal Mortality
    Enquiry)
  Peer review systems
  Utilization review
  Patient care profiles (Robins, Anthony and MacMillan,
    1993)
  Professional accreditation/examinations

---

process, such as Qualpacs, Monitor, and the CARE scheme (Wandelt and Ager, 1975; Goldstone, 1989; Research Unit of the Royal College of Physicians, 1992). Quality circles are also thought to be used widely (Hutchins, 1990).

The challenge is therefore to define the commonality between methods so that standards can be shared and training can be harmonized. Links between clinical audit and the delivery of care may be made more tangible by quality methods such as 'Collaborative care planning' and 'Anticipated recovery pathways'.

It is also worth mentioning the role of national audits, although this type of activity is limited to a minority of specialtes. The Confidential Enquiries into Maternal Mortality were the pathfinders in this field (UK Departments of Health, 1990). More recently, the NCEPOD (national confidential enquiry into perioperative deaths) project has become established (Campling, Devlin and Lunn, 1990) and appears to have the support of surgical colleagues. Similar audits have now been developed in other areas such as suicide and still-births/infant deaths.

National audits
- Mortality reviews
- Multisite audit projects
- Peer review

In the health care of elderly people, some large scale audit has begun and a national benchmarking audit exchange is being planned by the Royal College of Physicians. Additionally, systems such as peer review (Hopkins, 1990) and utilization review are also becoming established (Feldstein, Wickizer and Wheeler, 1988).

Organizational

Organizational methods are those that can be used right across organizations, involving all workers in some way. They may be managerial, quantitative or inspection systems.

Organizational activities
• Managerial
• Quantitative
• Inspection

Managerial systems. The most well known managerial methods is 'total quality management'. Often referred to as TQM (Oakland, 1989), it is also known as 'kaizen' and by a number of other synonyms. The principle here is that every aspect of the process of care is examined, that all appropriate workers are involved and that attention to the quality of care is a continuous activity.

A key element of success is instilling a quality 'culture' into the organization. This has an intuitive appeal, but changes in culture is one of the hardest changes for an organization to make. 'Every error is a jewel', – one of the catchphrases of TQM – encapsulates the idea that any lapse in the quality of care is an opportunity to improve it. This principle should be used in a non-punitive fashion throughout the organization. An allied concept is that of 'zero defects' – a more proactive stance towards getting health care right, first time, every time.

'Outcomes management' is a tantalizing method that seeks to base future care on the outcomes of previous care (Coles, 1990). However, routine systems for delivering timely outcomes information do not exist, and there is no consensus view on the outcomes that should be measured.

Finally, there is a group of methods concerned with serious adverse events which is referred to as 'critical incident' techniques (Flanagan, 1954). While a system such as this may have a valuable contribution, it cannot stand alone as a means to achieve high quality care.

Quantitative systems. The more quantitative approaches are exemplified by the King's Fund organizational audit programme, and a similar scheme in the South Western Region

(Shaw and Brooks, 1991). These concentrate on checking that resources and practices exist but they are uncertainly linked with the achievement of better patient outcomes. Neither should they be confused with a quality support system, such as British Standard 5750 (also known as ISO 9000, its international synonym) or a quality standard such as the Patient's Charter. Both of these are discussed below.

Inspection systems.   The final group of organization methods comprises those characterized by inspection and registration. These seek to improve the quality of care by external review, often with the threat of sanctions. Examples include the system of registration of nursing homes and inspection of training posts for doctors. Although these methods are a legitimate 'backstop', there is little evidence that these methods have any meaningful or sustained impact on the quality of care.

Tool 2: quality standards

Quality methods require standards of care against which staff can judge their work. Quality standards exist in many forms (Box 4.3) and their production is proliferating fast. Indeed a major tension is developing between locally set standards and nationally set standards. Although it was initially envisaged that most standards would be set locally, there is a growing recognition of the huge resources that might be wasted as a result of inevitable duplication. An emerging concept is that national clinical guidelines should be developed at a regional or local level by specialties with central facilitation.

Quality standards are usefully classified according to the classic audit framework (Donabedian, 1966), as those concerned with **structure** (such as facilities, staffing, training, procedures, etc.) and those concerned with **process** (the activities of care). In theory, standards should also exist for **outcome** but, as mentioned above, outcome measures remain crude and inadequate.

The mere existence of a quality standard cannot guarantee high quality care, since the adoption of a standard is likely to be a sterile exercise without a quality method to implement it. A selection of existing quality standards of relevance to the care of elderly people is shown in Box 4.3. Most of these are national level quality standards as little is known about what exists at local level.

Box 4.3   Quality standards

- Clinical: guidelines, policies and protocols
  Chiropody and podiatry practice (Society of Chiropodists, 1991)
  Clothing (Disabled Living Foundation, 1990)
  Stroke (Royal College of Physicians, 1989b; Effective Health Care, 1992; UK Stroke Audit Group, 1994)
  Pressure sores (King's Fund, 1989)
  Occupational therapy for consumers with physical disability
  Physiotherapy
  Speech therapy
- Non-clinical
  Patient's Charter
  Charter for disabled people using hospitals

Definitions
- Standard – must be done
- Guideline – should be done
- Option – could be done

The terminology surrounding quality standards is fuzzy. One person's standard might be another man's guideline. Eddy (1990) provides a helpful definition – standards are what **must** be done, guidelines are what **should** be done, and options are what **can** be done. Thus, a standard would legitimately be based upon the results of a rigorous trial, guidelines upon other evidence, and an option on observed practice.

There are several clinical guidelines that are relevant to the care of elderly people. The College of Occupational Therapists (1991), the Chartered Society of Physiotherapy (1990) and the College of Speech and Language Therapists (1991) have all produced professional standards, and a *Charter for Disabled People using Hospital* was published in 1992 (Royal College of Physicians, 1992). There are also clinical guidelines for the assessment of disability among elderly people and day hospital care (Research Unit the Royal College of Physicians/British Geriatrics Society, 1992, 1994). Many more standards are in existence.

Tool 3: quality measures

The development of valid and reliable quality measures is central to real progress in improving the quality of care. Measures are needed for two main purposes: first, to categorize groups of similar patients to allow valid comparisons (**case mix** measures); second, to measure the health of patients and how it is changed by health interventions (**outcome** measures). A number of candidate measures exist (Box 4.4), and there is a national outcomes clearing house, which aims to facilitate development in this area (Nuffield Institute for Health, 1992). However, there is no real consensus on how outcomes should be measured.

Box 4.4   Quality measures

- Case mix groups and systems
  Diagnosis related groups (DRGs) (Fetter *et al.*, 1980)
  Health related groups (HRGs) (National Casemix Office, 1992)
  Resource utilization groups (RUGs) (Fries and Cooney, 1985)
  Coded disease staging (Gonnella, Hornbrook and Louis, 1984)
  Computerized Severity Index (CSI) (Horn and Horn, 1986)
  Medical Illness Grouping System (Medisgroups) (Brewster *et al.*, 1985)
  Patient Management Categories (PMCs) (Young, 1984)
- Severity ratings
  APACHE II (Knaus *et al.*, 1985)
  Rankin Score (Rankin, 1957)
- Potential outcome measures
  Goal attainment scaling (Stolee *et al.*, 1992)
  Quality of life measures:
     Philadelphia Geriatric Center Morale Scale (Powell-Lawton, 1975)
  Multidimensional health profiles:
     Nottingham Health Profile (Hunt *et al.*, 1980)
     SF36 (Garratt *et al.*, 1993)
  Disability measures:
     Barthel ADL Index (Collin *et al.*, 1988)
     Nottingham Extended ADL scale (Nouri and Lincoln, 1987)
  Handicap measure (Harwood *et al.*, 1994)
- Patient satisfaction
  Several approaches (Fitzpatrick, 1990)

Practice point
Quality support systems do not guarantee high quality

Tool 4: quality support systems

The success of quality methods depends both on staff factors, such as enthusiasm and motivation, and organizational factors, such as the quality support systems. It has become clear that sustained success is strongly reliant on the latter. For example, when medical audit began, doctors spent time inappropriately retrieving case notes. In many units, this is now carried out by audit staff. The fact that a high proportion of case notes cannot be found implies that there is a need for a further step of improvement in medical record systems.

A quality support system may arise to service a particular quality initiative. There is also increasing interest in externally validated quality support systems such as BS 5750, which is becoming popular in the health service. This British standard requires the organization to put in place a system to prove what has been done in pursuit of quality; there is no guarantee that any level of quality has been achieved.

Practice point
• Use the tool to suit the job
• Use more than one tool

Using the toolbox

The extent to which the different quality tools are used will vary according to circumstances. For instance, outcome measures are poorly developed at present and this limits the extent to which a quality method such as outcomes management can be used. On the other hand, the use of some quality methods is intimately bound up with the setting of quality standards, such as in the Dynamic Standard Setting System (DySSSy) initiated by the Royal College of Nursing (1990). In general, any proposal for quality work that only uses one tool should not be pursued seriously.

Practice point
Seven questions to judge a quality proposal

Any suggested quality initiative should be viewed from several perspectives to assess its acceptability and likelihood of success. Here are some questions to ask about any quality proposal:

• Who are the beneficiaries? Is it concerned with purchasers, providers or consumers?
• Does it involve the whole organization, a particular service or a single profession?
• Have other relevant care sectors, such as primary, tertiary or community care, been considered?

- Does it deal with structure, process, outcome or patient satisfaction?
- Is the proposal punitive, facilitatory or educational?
- What is the evidence of commitment behind the proposal? Is it just 'window dressing', or it is backed with concrete resources such as money, incentives, information and training for staff? Will staff have time to participate?
- Are there appropriate links with accreditation systems, continuing professional education, and research and development?

Thus, a quality proposal needs to be coherent and comprehensive. Special issues, such as system logistics, team-working and boundaries of care, should be tackled. There is a strong sense that these are the areas where 'things go wrong'. The proposal should include some estimate of the value for money that the initiative might deliver. There is a lot of cynicism about 'the cost of quality' but the costs of low quality care may be enormous for the service, the patient and carers. Consider the costs of an adverse event such as a pressure sore, or the costs of poor liaison with community services resulting in wasted bed-days.

A LOOK TO THE FUTURE

This section suggests how the quality movement might change in the future and what new directions it might take. The three important trends discussed are:

- Management strengthening
- Business ideas
- Heightened consumer focus.

> **Main trends**
> - Management strengthening
> - Business ideas
> - Increased consumer focus

Management strengthening

It seems likely that the management of the health system will be greatly strengthened. More and more managers are receiving appropriate training and there are several government backed initiatives to ensure this is the case. This will have the effect of providing a constant organizational backdrop dedicated to quality and complementing professional activities.

Business ideas

There is likely to be further transfer of ideas from commerce to public sectors such as the health service.

Use of the marketing concept

This refers to the concept of succeeding by discerning the needs of customers and seeking to fulfil them. It has formed the basis of success for many organizations and is likely to influence the health service, particularly as the primacy of the consumer becomes recognized.

Accounting development

Companies are required by law to produce accounts using traditional accounting methods. However, there are moves towards more appropriate ways of assigning costs, particularly in relation to the activities of the organization and its strategy. Given the very poor understanding of the cost base of the health service, it is hoped that such thinking might be incorporated into health service accounting development. This would affect the quality movement by clarifying the costs of quality.

Appropriate use of information technology (IT)

The management of information has been harnessed to revolutionize many aspects of industry. Clearly, such expertise needs to percolate through to the health system where the information base is very weak. The development of an electronic patient record will bear heavy responsibility for fully realizing this potential.

Heightened consumer focus

The involvement of consumers in health care is likely to rise rapidly. This will further reinforce the pressure for high quality care and help to define the characteristics of high quality care more clearly.

It will probably occur at several levels. At the level of the individual patient, we may see more concern with communication and joint decision making, possibly assisted by patient information in different formats. At the level of the unit or service, we may see the emergence of more user groups. At the population level, the need for more explicit rationing implies the need for purchasers to engage more closely with the local population. This has already been encouraged by the clear new responsibilities of purchasers to the needs of the local population, by central initiatives such as *Local voices. The views of local people in purchasing for health* (NHS Management Executive, 1992) and by diverse local experiments in this area (Bowling, 1993).

CONCLUSION

This chapter has presented a strategic level view of the quality movement in health services. It showed how quality has diffused from product manufacture, to services, then public services before becoming rooted in the health service. In the health sector, three broad principles have emerged – clarity about the meaning of high quality care, the different dimensions of quality in health care, and the role of quality cycles. The concept of the quality toolbox provides a way of considering the wide variety of quality activities that are now being undertaken, distinguishing quality methods, standards, measures and support systems. This assists us in making choices about how to tackle quality. One feature of quality that has emerged is that success depends on people. Thus, the management of the health service must ensure that staff are supported by an organization, system and resources to succeed. Enormous progress has already been made by the quality movement in the health service. It seems likely that the momentum will be maintained.

REFERENCES

Age Concern (1994) *Gold standards*, Age Concern, London.

Bank, J. (1992) *The essence of total quality management*, Prentice Hall, London.

Bowling, A. (1993) *What people are saying about prioritising health services*, King's Fund Centre, London.

Brewster, A.C., Karlin, B.G., Hyde, L.A. *et al.* (1985) MEDISGROUPS: a clinically based approach to classifying hospital patients at admission. *Inquiry*, **12**, 377–87.

Brook, R.H. and Kosecoff, J.B. (1988) Commentary: competition and quality. *Health Affairs*, **7**, 150–61.

Campling, E.A., Devlin, H.B. and Lunn, J.N. (1990) *Report of the national confidential enquiry into perioperative deaths* (NCEPOD), NCEPOD, London.

Chartered Society of Physiotherapy (1990) *Standards of physiotherapy practice pack*, CSP, London.

Chase, R.B. and Aquilano, NJ. (1989) *Production and operations management: a life cycle approach*, Irwin, Homewood.

Coles, J. (1990) Outcomes management and performance indicators, in *Measuring the outcomes of medical care* (eds A. Hopkins, and D. Costain), Royal College of Physicians and King's Fund Centre, London.

College of Occupational Therapists (1991) *Occupational therapy for consumers with physical disabilities*, COT, London.

College of Speech and Language Therapists (1991) *Communicating quality: professional standards for speech and language therapists*, CSLT, London.

Collin, C., Wade, D.T., Davies, S. and Horne, V. (1988) The Barthel ADL Index: a reliability study. *International Disability Studies*, **10**, 1–3.

Department of Health (1989) *Working for patients*, HMSO, London.

Department of Health (1991) *Patient's Charter. Raising the standard*, HMSO, London.

Department of Health (1993a) *Clinical audit. Meeting and improving standards in health care*, DoH, London.

Department of Health (1993b) *Research for health*, DoH, London.

Disabled Living Foundation (1990) *Clothing: a quality issue. Provision of clothing for people living in NHS hospitals and units*, King's Fund/Royal College of Nursing, London.

Donabedian, A. (1966) Evaluating the quality of medical care. *Millbank Memorial Fund Quarterly*, **44**(Supplement), 166–206.

Eddy, D.M. (1990) Clinical decision-making: from theory to practice. Practice policies – what are they? *Journal of the American Medical Association*, **263**, 877–80.

Effective Health Care (1992) Stroke rehabilitation, School of Public Health, University of Leeds, Leeds.

Feldstein, P.J., Wickizer, T.M. and Wheeler, J.R.C. (1988) Private cost containment. The effects of utilization review programs in health care use and expenditure. *New England Journal of Medicine*, **318**, 1310–14.

Fetter, R.B., Shin, Y., Freeman, J. *et al.* (1980) Case-mix definition by diagnosis-related groups. *Medical Care*, **18**(Supplement), 1–53.

Fitzpatrick, R. (1990) Measurement of patient satisfaction, in *Measuring the outcomes of medical care* (eds A. Hopkins, and D. Costain), Royal College of Physicians and King's Fund Centre, London.

Flanagan, J.C. (1954) The critical incident technique. *Psychology Bulletin*, **51**, 327–58.

Fries, B.E. and Cooney, L.M. (1985) Resource Utilisation Groups: a patient classification system for long-term care. *Medical Care*, **23**, 100–122.

Garratt, A., Ruta, D., Abdalla, M.I. *et al.* (1993) The SF36 health survey questionnaire: an outcome measure suitable for routine use within the NHS? *British Medical Journal*, **306**, 1440–4.

Garvin, D.A. (1987) Competing on the eight dimensions of quality, *Harvard Business Review*, **Nov/Dec**.

Ghobadian, A. and Speller, S. (1994) Gurus for quality: a framework for comparison. *Total Quality Management*, **5**, 53–69.

Goldstone, L.A. (1989) *Monitor: an index of the quality of nursing care for acute medical and surgical wards*, Newcastle upon Tyne Polytechnic Products Ltd, Newcastle upon Tyne.

Gonnella, J.S., Hornbrook, M.C. and Louis D.Z. (1984) Staging of disease: a casemix measurement. *Journal of the American Medical Association*, **251**, 637–46.

Harwood, R., Rogers, A., Dickinson, E. and Ebrahim, S. (1994) Measuring handicap: the London handicap scale, a new outcome measure for chronic disease. *Quality in Health Care*, **3**, 11–16.

Hopkins, A. (1990) *Measuring the quality of medical care*, Royal College of Physicians, London.

Horn, S.D. and Horn, R.A. (1986) The computerised severity index: a new tool for case-mix management. *Journal of Medical Systems*, **10**, 73–8.

Hunt, S.M., McKenna, J., Backett, E.M. *et al.* (1980) A quantitative approach to perceived health status: a validation study. *Journal of Epidemiology and Community Health*, **34**, 281–6.

Hutchins, D. (1990) *In pursuit of quality*, Pitman, London.

Institute of Health Service Managers (1989) *Management of quality*, IHSM, London.

Johnson, G. and Scholes, K. (1993) *Exploring corporate strategy*, Prentice Hall, London.

King's Fund (1989) *The prevention and management of pressure sores within health districts*, King's Fund Centre, London.

Knaus, W.A., Draper, E.A., Wagner, D.P. and Zimmerman, J.E. (1985) APACHE II: a severity of disease classification system. *Critical Care Medicine*, **13**, 818–29.

Lorenz, B. (1993) The side-effects of a cure-all approach. *Financial Times*, 2 April, 11.

Maxwell, R.J. (1994) Quality assessment in health. *British Medical Journal*, **288**, 1470–2.

National Casemix Office (1992) *Definitions manual for health care resource groups*, NCMO, Winchester.

NHS Management Executive (1992) *Local voices. The views of local people in purchasing for health*, Department of Health, London.

NHS Management Executive (1993) *A to Z of quality: a guide to quality initiatives in the NHS*, HMSO, London.

Nouri, F. and Lincoln, N.B. (1987) An extended activities of daily living scale for stroke patients. *Clinical Rehabilitation*, **1**, 301–5.

Nuffield Institute for Health (1992) *Outcome Briefing*, issue 1, Nuffield Institute for Health, Leeds.

Oakland, J.S. (1989) *Total quality management*, Butterworth, Oxford.

Parasuraman, A., Zeithaml, V.A. and Berry, L.L. (1985) A conceptual model of service quality and its implications for future research. *Journal of Marketing*, **49**, 41–50.

Powell-Lawton, M. (1975) The Philadelphia Geriatric Center Morale Scale. *Journal of Gerontology*, **30**, 85–9.

Rankin, J. (1957) Cerebrovascular accidents in patients over the age of 60. II: prognosis. *Scottish Medical Journal*, **2**, 200.

Relman, A.S. (1988) Assessment and accountability: the third revolution. *New England Journal of Medicine*, **319**, 1220–8.

Research Unit of the Royal College of Physicians (1992) *The RCP CARE (continuous assessment, review and evaluation) scheme*, Royal College of Physicians, London.

Research Unit of the Royal College of Physicians and the British Geriatrics Society (1992) *Standardised assessment scales for elderly people*, Royal College of Physicians, London.

Research Unit of the Royal College of Physicians and the British Geriatrics Society (1994) *Geriatric day hospitals. Their role and guidelines for good practice*, Royal College of Physicians, London.

Robins, J.B., Anthony, G.S. and MacMillan, R. (1993) Profiles of patient care. *Hospital Update Plus*, **June**, 97S–101S.

Royal College of Nursing (1990) *Dynamic standard setting system (DySSSy)*, RCN, Scutari Press, London.

Royal College of Physicians (1989a) *Medical Audit. A first report. What, why and how?* RCP, London.

Royal College of Physicians (1989b) *The management of stroke*, RCP, London.

Royal College of Physicians (1992) *A charter for disabled people using hospitals*, RCP, London.

Royal College of Physicians (1993) *Medical Audit. A second report*, RCP, London.

Scottish Office (1993) *Clinical Guidelines*, HMSO, Edinburgh.

Shaw, C.D. and Brooks, T.E. (1991) Health services accreditation in the United Kingdom. *Quality Assurance in Health Care*, **3**, 133–40.

Social Services Inspectorate (1990) *Caring for quality. Guidance of standards for residential homes for elderly people*, HMSO, London.

Society of Chiropodists (1991) *Guidelines on standards of chiropody and podiatry practice*, Society of Chiropodists, London.

Stolee, P., Rockwood, K., Fox, R. and Streiner, D.L. (1992) The use of goal attainment scaling in a geriatric care setting. *Journal of the American Geriatric Society*, **40**, 574–8.

UK Departments of Health (1991) *Report on confidential enquiries into maternal deaths in the UK 1985–7*, HMSO, London.

UK Stroke Audit Group (1994) *An audit protocol for stroke patients*, Royal College of Physicians, London.

Wandelt, M.A. and Ager, J. (1975) *Quality patient care scale*, Wayne State University, Detroit.

Young, W.A. (1984) Incorporating severity of illness and comorbidity in case-mix measurement. *Health Care Financing Revolution*, **6**(Supplement), 23–31.

Part Two
Sectors

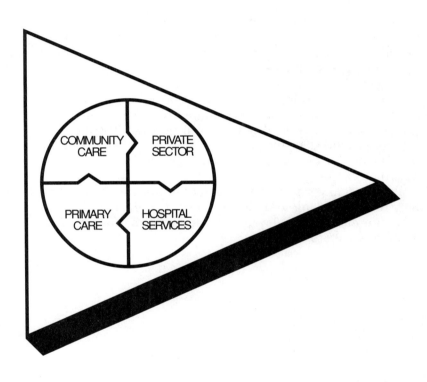

EDITORS' INTRODUCTION TO PART TWO

The first slice across the health care of elderly people is across the different sectors of care. Successful care is often dependent on the relationships between different care sectors. This is because elderly people often have complex needs and chronic diseases punctuated by episodes of acute events. Despite this the interface between 'health' and 'social' care is controversial, often hazy and constantly shifting. As we have seen in Part One, the activities of the different sectors and the relationships between them are subject to wide influences. Part Two shows the response in the different sectors.

This part aims to show the issues and activities in the main care sectors, in particular by looking at the service developments and quality initiatives that are occurring. Although there is no specific chapter concerned with the contribution of the voluntary sector, this is more a symptom of lack of space rather than deliberate exclusion. We anticipate that reading Part Two will give an understanding of some of the key factors of concern to the different sectors that will affect the quality of care.

Chapter 5, on Primary health care, provides a practical approach to quality. The stages described are of relevance and could be applied in any setting of care.

Chapter 6 tackles quality in community care by describing what led to the current policy and the challenges that need to be solved to make it work.

Chapter 7 takes us through the role of the private sector, concentrating on quality initiatives in response to the needs of purchasers and regulators but with a sophisticated eye to the demands of users.

Chapter 8 looks at hospital services. It aims to demystify what hospitals are trying to do and how they are trying to do it. The role of clinical audit is explained in detail.

By the end of Part Two, the reader will be aware of the key issues and activities in the dominant sectors of care.

Primary health care for elderly people 5

Richard Baker

EDITORS' INTRODUCTION

This chapter opens the part of the book that considers four different sectors of care. It present a practical approach to developing high quality primary care for elderly people, taking the reader through the basic stages. The importance attached to the development of primary care is symbolized by this chapter.

The chapter is made up of five main parts. First, Dr Baker considers why elderly people should be considered as a special group in primary care, and makes a very good case for this on the basis of team-based care, the primary care implications of an ageing population and the fact that there is ample scope for improving the quality of care. Next follow four sections that explain a step by step approach to quality: plan development; agreeing priorities; implementation; and monitoring. These steps are discussed in the context of primary care, but the essential themes have great relevance to the other sectors of care. For example, practical ways of assessing patient opinions and approaches to implementation are given.

Although this chapter is about making quality work, Dr Baker does not forget that all services are delivered by organizations that are managed. Thus, the approach he advocates links with general management theory and there is an emphasis on involving management in implementation.

This chapter will give readers a practical overview of thinking in primary care and an understanding of the practical stages of quality that can be applied in any situation. The closest analogy to the challenge of quality in primary care is that in community care, and Chapter 6 outlines some of the

Key topics
- Elderly people as a special group
- Developing a quality plan
- Prioritization
- Carrying out the plan
- Monitoring

Quality Care for Elderly People. Edited by Peter P. Mayer, Edward J. Dickinson and Martin Sandler. Published in 1997 by Chapman & Hall, London. ISBN 0 412 61830 3

changes required in this sector. Dr Baker indicates the need for primary care to respond to health care in the residential setting, and it is interesting to compare this with developments in the private sector (Chapter 7).

INTRODUCTION

Case study 5.1.
Mrs T., a 74-year-old woman, was fitted in to see me in surgery when her usual doctor was not available. She had a cold and some aches and pains. There was not much to find on examination, apart from her long-standing osteoarthritis. Throughout the consultation she appeared anxious and sorry for herself.

'You don't sound very happy' I said.

She agreed, and began to cry, saying she had not meant that to happen. She told me that her husband was restless at night and kept her awake, and that her son had committed suicide five years before, following the death of his wife a year before that. Then she expressed her worries about her husband, who had attempted suicide twice in the past 18 months, although he had promised not to try it again. We talked. She had brought up six children, worked most of her life, and been the dependable source of support to her family throughout. Together we agreed how much she had achieved in her life and by the end of the consultation she was more cheerful and optimistic. [Details modified to protect confidentiality].

The complexity of primary health care for elderly people should not be underestimated. They often have several clinical conditions, but also a blend of family, social and personal histories which may, from the clinical point of view, be equally important in decisions about their management.

The assurance of quality in these circumstances is challenging. In the case of Mrs T., (Case study 5.1) a prescription for any one of three possible diagnoses might have been considered (respiratory infection, osteoarthritis, depression), but the opportunity to reflect and recognition of how she had supported her family proved more valuable.

On other occasions, early diagnosis is critical. For patients with chronic diseases, long-term anticipatory monitoring based on clinical practice guidelines or other authoritative sources of research evidence is undertaken to prevent complications and maintain independence. It follows that quality assurance strategies for use in primary health care must take into account the various needs both of different patient groups and individual patients.

Health care teams can discharge their burden of responsibility to elderly patients by adopting a few simple measures which together constitute systematic management combined with the essential humane flexibility required by elderly patients. This chapter discusses the steps that can be taken by primary health care teams to ensure that elderly patients receive effective and appropriate care.

ELDERLY PEOPLE AS A PATIENT SUB-GROUP

The overwhelming majority of health care received by elderly people is provided by different members of primary health care teams. These teams are the first point of contact when symptoms arise, deal directly with the majority of presenting complaints and refer on to secondary care those who need specialist help. Furthermore, primary health care services both provide support to those who are chronically ill or disabled, and are responsible for assessing the need for support of patients and their carers. Thus, the quality of care received by elderly patients and the quality of life of those who become ill will depend, in large measure, on the primary health care team.

There is a growing body of evidence that the primary health care of elderly patients and the support of their carers could be improved. Admittedly, this does not necessarily mean that elderly patients are receiving care that is in some way worse than that given to those in other age groups, but it does indicate that there are particular problems in the care of elderly people that require specific attention.

The findings are consistent across a range of clinical conditions and also apply to patients with chronic disabilities or who are dependent upon social support. Furthermore, increasing life expectancy and the growing number of elderly people have implications for primary health care. These issues will be illustrated by reference to a few selected research studies.

In a study of the diagnosis and management of depression in elderly patients MacDonald (1986) found that although general practitioners (GPs) did not miss many cases of depression, they were unlikely to institute vigorous treatment. The overall rate of prescriptions for antidepressant drugs was low, and referral to other agencies, such as social serv-

Why a special case?
- Team-based care
- Scope for improvement
- Primary care implications of an ageing population
- The impact of disability

Possible improvement areas
- Treatment of depression
- Treatment of hypertension
- Management of diabetes

ices, was uncommon. In a survey of the management of elderly patients with hypertension, GPs appeared to be unclear about appropriate management: few reported checking standing blood pressure, despite the high prevalence of postural hypotension in the elderly; and one-third would not treat isolated systolic hypertension (Fotherby, Harper and Potter 1992). It is also necessary to modify our views and management of some diseases in response to the changing age pattern of the population and the availability of new, more effective treatments. In a commentary on the management of elderly patients with diabetes, Sinclair and Barnett (1993) point out that because of increasing life expectancy, many elderly diabetic patients now live long enough to suffer from potentially preventable complications such as blindness and foot ulceration. The established view has been that the aim of care in elderly diabetics is to avoid hypoglycaemia and symptoms of hyperglycaemia, but this limited view now needs to be challenged.

Dependent elderly people are a specific group with particular needs. In a survey of patients over the age of 70 in two general practices in South Wales, it was found that 24% were unable to go shopping, 7.7% were unable to climb stairs, 6% were unable to walk out of doors and 1.3% were unable to walk indoors (Vetter, Lewis and Llewellyn, 1992). The authors of this study found that one person, usually a daughter or spouse, made the major contribution to caring.

In a study of elderly patients who had to be unexpectedly readmitted to hospital following discharge, carers complained about the effect on their own health of caring for their relative and the many difficulties and frustrations they faced (Williams and Fitton, 1991). Seventy-one per cent of the carers in the readmitted group were involved in at least one intimate task such as dressing, bathing or coping with incontinence. They were also more likely than the carers of patients who did not have to be readmitted to be involved in dressing the elderly patients, getting them up in the morning and putting them to bed at night. Carers of patients who had to be readmitted pointed to frustration caused by the continuous pressure of the needs of the people in their care (44%) and dissatisfaction with medical care in hospital (29%).

In an audit of the support given by the primary care team to the carers of elderly demented patients, it was found that lay carers lacked knowledge and had unmet needs (Philp and Young, 1988). The unmet needs included support from day

---

Impact of disability
- Functional limitation
- Carer strain
- Responsibility for long-term care residents

centres, respite admissions, attendance allowance, community nursing services and relative support groups. These were provided during the course of the audit to most of those in need, and a repeat survey indicated that more of the needs had been met.

Elderly dependent patients in residential homes represent a particularly dependent subgroup, and the majority of their medical care is provided by the primary care team. In a comparison of the number and level of dependency of patients in residential care in 1979 with 1990 in Leicestershire, there was a 30% increase in the number of dependent patients, while dependency levels rose significantly, most steeply in the private sector (Stern, Jagger and Clark, 1993). The findings reflect the transfer of responsibility between the different forms of provision for long-term dependent elderly patients that has taken place.

A PLAN OF ACTION

A team of health professionals caring for elderly people needs a policy or plan for the quality assurance and improvement of the care it provides. Many teams will now have long-term and short-term business plans, although these may often focus only on organizational factors rather than clinical issues. The development of services for elderly people by primary health care teams should be one part of these long-term plans. An idealized diagram of such a plan is shown in Figure 5.1, which assumes a multidisciplinary team that includes doctors, nurses and administrative staff, responsible for a defined and identifiable group of patients. The diagram is a development of a model for the management of audit by the primary health care team (Hearnshaw, 1993). The team has a specific structure responsible for overall team management. The precise constitution of this management group will vary according to the size of the health care team and the organization of the health service in which it is situated. Nevertheless, the broad principles are likely to be applicable in the majority of primary health care settings.

Objectives

The first stage in developing a plan for the care of elderly patients is for the team to agree a common core of objectives. It is unlikely that care will be effective unless the team has a

---

Objectives
Objectives should be:
- based on shared values
- agreed
- worthwhile
- communicated

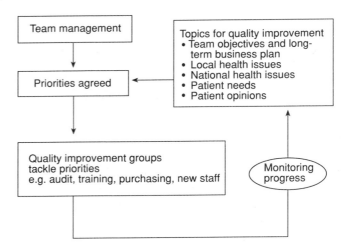

Figure 5.1 A primary health care team quality improvement plan.

set of shared values about the importance of care for this group and an understanding of the different contributions that can be made by each professional in the team. The team also needs to decide whether it feels sufficiently strongly about the quality of care given to elderly patients, and the process of agreeing objectives will enable these issues to be aired adequately. Agreement can only be reached after discussion and shared understanding, which may take place formally or informally as part of team meetings. Different teams will have different ways of working together, but even in the smallest team co-operation will be impossible without communication. In the absence of effective systems of communication, such as regular team meetings, agreement about developing care is left to chance. In teams that do have difficulties, facilitators can help the negotiation of agreement. Many health authorities now employ facilitators to support developments in primary health care, and others work as part of audit groups and therefore this type of practical assistance is widely available.

Local priorities and national clinical guidelines

There may already be established priorities for health care in the locality. The local health authority may be seeking to improve care of patients with diabetes or may have chosen to set goals for the care of dependent elderly people in the

Practice point
Always consider:
- local priorities
- local need
- local culture
- national priorities
- national guidelines

community. In some areas there may be a large number of elderly living alone and in need of support (Forbes, 1996); in deprived areas some elderly people may be particularly poor and in need of assessment and advice about the financial allowances that may be available to them (Teale, 1996). In areas with a high proportion of patients from ethnic groups there may be problems arising from language and cultural differences (Ebrahim, 1996).

In the past few years it has been increasingly recognized that clinical practice is often not in accord with current best research evidence. Clinical practice guidelines, defined as 'systematically developed statements to assist practitioner and patient decisions about appropriate health care for specific clinical circumstances' (Institute of Medicine, 1992) are seen as one method for resolving this problem (NHS Executive, 1996). Evidence-based medicine is a related approach in which the practitioner is encouraged to track down, critically appraise and incorporate the best possible evidence into practice (Sackett and Rosenberg, 1995) and even in general practice the majority of clinical interventions can be related to good quality research evidence (Gill *et al.*, 1996).

The development of scientifically valid guidelines is a complex task which can only be adequately undertaken by those with the necessary expertise and resources, but examples for several common clinical conditions are becoming available (Eccles *et al.*, 1996). It has been suggested that the most efficient way to employ guidelines is for national agencies to develop them using appropriate methods. Local practice teams, or local health authorities or trusts, can then adapt the guidelines to meet local circumstances and implement them in practice (Royal College of General Practitioners, 1995). Teams seeking to improve the quality of care of elderly people will need to identify relevant clinical guidelines and use effective methods for incorporating the recommendations they contain into daily practice.

Patient needs

There are very few examples of organized needs assessment being undertaken by primary health care teams for the purposes of organizing care to meet the needs of their elderly patients. A minimum data set for planning the care of the elderly has been described (Jachuck and Mulcaahy, 1987) and a simple and practical approach has been reported (Murray *et al.*, 1994). However, the purpose of identifying

> **Practice point**
> Identifying priorities: need **plus** deficient care

aspects of care to which the team should direct particular attention is not merely about needs assessment. It is also necessary to identify aspects of care that are deficient in some way and which, in consequence, should be priorities for quality improvement.

Information about the needs of patients is readily available from a number of sources. Members of the team will be only too well aware of many of the gaps in quality that come to their attention. For example, it may be found that a patient has not been visited by a nurse because the message from the doctor was not transmitted by the administrative staff, or a patient has been admitted to hospital because of a drug interaction. It is important to learn from such problems, and significant event audit can be one approach (Pringle *et al.*, 1995). One source of data is the practice disease register. A basic preliminary is to ascertain the number of elderly patients registered with the practice. However, information is also needed about the health and social circumstances of these patients. Computerized practices will easily be able to identify the number of elderly patients with diabetes, hypertension or other chronic disorders. Some practices may have also recorded information about patients who are dependent or living alone, and again this would be useful background data. A variety of sociodemographic information may also be available from the local health authority, such as underprivileged area scores (Jarman, 1985), and hospital admission rates. The team should attempt to calculate the number of elderly people living in residential and nursing homes, as they form a particularly dependent group.

> **Ways of understanding needs**
> - Team knowledge
> - Practice disease register
> - Local health authority data

Patient opinions

The views of elderly people themselves must not be forgotten. The conduct of surveys of patient opinion is now common. However, there are no standardized instruments for use with an elderly patient population to enable them to pinpoint aspects of care that are unsatisfactory, and a team wishing to survey the opinion of its elderly patients may need to design its own survey.

The traditional method is a paper and pencil questionnaire. This can reveal important concerns, but it does have a number of disadvantages. The first is that it takes time and skill to develop a questionnaire that is meaningful. There are numerous examples of poor questionnaires that produce only misleading information. Secondly, the questionnaire may only identify a limited range of information. Nevertheless, questionnaires can be helpful, and there are examples of instruments for obtaining general information that have been tested for reliability and validity, and can be completed by an elderly patient group (Baker and Whitfield, 1992).

Elderly people are more likely to experience higher levels of continuity of care and studies confirm that this is an important feature in determining patient satisfaction (Baker, 1996). When several variables explaining levels of satisfaction were taken into account, satisfaction was found to fall with increasing patient age, unless the practice operated a personal list system, in which case satisfaction increased with patient age (Baker and Streatfield, 1995). Assistance in the design of a questionnaire may be obtained from the local health authority or clinical audit group. Teams planning to use a questionnaire would be wise to consult these sources of support.

There are other means of collecting information from patients. Qualitative interviews of specific patient groups can be revealing. It should be remembered that interviewing is just as skilled a process as questionnaire design. The employment of an expert in interview techniques can be worthwhile, although it is expensive and likely to be beyond the means of most practices.

Patient participation groups are another approach, although they do tend to be unrepresentative. One advantage of patient participation groups is that they can harness the ability of the local patient community to offer support to dependent people, for example by providing prescription collection services, transport services or visiting the house bound elderly. Focus groups offer an alternative method for surveying opinions (Krueger, 1988). The practice invites six or eight elderly patients to attend a group and the group facilitator asks them a small number of questions about the quality of services they have received. The facilitator should be skilled and the discussions should be recorded on tape for transcription and analysis. Focus groups can be convenient for collecting information, although it should be acknowledged that, as with other methods, the novice should seek support and guidance.

A simple system that should be used by any practice team is the collection of unsolicited comments from patients as they use the services (Baker *et al.*, 1994). Patients often make comments about delays in seeing the doctor, difficulties they

Practice point
Other ways of obtaining patient opinions:
- special interviews
- patient participation groups
- focus groups
- collecting unsolicited comments

experienced in getting through to the surgery on the telephone, the interpersonal skills of different members of the practice team, and so forth. On most occasions these remarks are largely ignored. However, systematically collecting this live information will soon give the team insight into how patients experience the service.

AGREEING PRIORITIES

Resources for agreeing priorities
- Local and national priorities
- Needs
- Views of patients

Practice point
Top priorities should:
- affect many people
- be amenable to improvement
- be worthwhile in patient outcomes
- fit with team care purpose

The above discussions make clear that there is an enormous range of factors that practices could take into account in developing their services for elderly people. They include local priorities, national guidelines, patients' needs and their satisfaction with care. In reality it is unlikely that all these issues would be addressed simultaneously, but nevertheless, in order to cope, the team must prioritize the issues that have been identified.

Prioritization will depend on whether each problem has a significant impact on patient morbidity or mortality, affects large numbers of patients, is amenable to strategies that the primary health care team might employ, and is supported by convincing research evidence that indicates that it would be worth the investment of time and energy in terms of bringing about benefits in patient care. The issues must also be reviewed in the light of the team's overall objectives, and will therefore need consideration by all team members.

Elderly patients, like all other patients, require a service that takes account of their individual needs, their level of understanding, and their dependence on a continuing and personal relationship with the health professional, which enables them to express all their concerns and feel that they are understood. It is for this reason that emphasis has been placed in this discussion on the need to listen directly to patient opinions and respond to them in the planning of care. If the appointment system is chaotic, the length of appointments short and consultations rushed, it is unlikely that elderly patients will be able to use the service effectively or express their deepest concerns in the consulting room.

Practice point
Assemble quality improvement groups for specific tasks

IMPLEMENTING THE PLAN

Having selected a set of priorities, a strategy must be devised for each one. The model in Figure 5.1 assumes that a number of groups will be convened and given responsibility for tackling one or more of the issues of concern. The details of this arrangement will vary according to the size and composition of the team, but in most circumstances delegation linked to a requirement for reporting back to team management is likely to be the most appropriate arrangement. The membership of the quality improvement groups will depend on the topic in question, for example, a group given the task of improving the quality of care of patients with varicose ulcers might include a GP, a community nurse and perhaps also a health visitor or community pharmacist (Baker *et al.*, 1995).

The methods that can be used by the quality improvement groups include clinical audit, new changes to the organization of services, education, reminders, the introduction of clinical practice guidelines (Grimshaw and Russell, 1994), purchasing services from secondary care, team building and many others. A variety of strategies have been shown to be effective in changing clinical performance, but no strategy is always effective, and much appears to depend on the nature of the change and the clinical setting concerned (Davis *et al.*, 1995; Grol, 1992). The way forward for each practice team is not in selecting one or other of these as the 'best buy', but in choosing the most appropriate strategy for the problem (Robertson *et al.*, 1996). The team will initially need to consider whether improvement requires negotiation between the practice and other services, for example over the appointment of an additional social worker or health visitor, or whether representation will need to be made to particular bodies, such as those concerned with the allocation of elderly people to residential homes or the level of communication with the local hospital. These are examples of change being possible only through collaboration with those external to the practice team.

Contracting for secondary care as part of fundholding or through health commissions is an example in which the primary health care team has been allocated a particularly powerful position. Secondary care providers may have a different view of their services to those of their patients or GP customers (Hicks and Baker, 1991). For example, they may feel that their service for patients with cataracts is excellent, including the use of new surgical procedures, whereas patients and their GPs may feel that the delay for appointments is unacceptable, and that the provision of low vision aids is completely inadequate. Purchasing offers an opportunity to redress the balance between 'hi-tech' care and the less glam-

Options for implementing an improved care strategy
• Clinical audit
• Service reorganization
• Clinical guidelines
• New care purchases
• Team building
• Others

Purchasing can bring together the opposite views of primary care and secondary care.

Case study 5.2   Quality improvement in the management of varicose ulcers

Setting
A single primary health care team in the UK. There are 12 000 registered patients, six GPs, and a full complement of nursing and administrative staff.

The problem
The nurses reported that the care of elderly patients with varicose ulcers was taking up a lot of their time and that the patients did not seem to improve.

The plan
A GP and a nurse identified all patients with a varicose ulcer and reviewed the medical records of each. Sixteen patients were found. Many had had their ulcers for several years. All patients saw a GP and a nurse regularly, but the dressings and medication being used were haphazard, with no clear management plan for any patient.

The solution
The audit/quality improvement group recommended that there should be regular consultation between the GP and nurse responsible for each patient so that a management plan could be agreed and modified according to the progress of the patient.

The outcome
One year later, the group once again reviewed the records of patients identified as having varicose ulcers. Of the 18 patients that were found on this occasion, the ulcers of seven patients had healed, and a further seven were improving. Given that many of the ulcers had been present for years, the change was startling. The reviews of each patient had led to more systematic management, including referral of patients for vascular surgery and grafting.

Conclusion
A systematic approach and effective communication in the team can lead to important improvements in health for some patients. The audit was easy to undertake and involved very little time.

orous and neglected basics that are so important to many patients.

If the quality improvement group feels that the resolution of the problem lies in the hands of the team members, the strategies adopted will depend upon the size of the team, the resources available, the particular topics under consideration, and other long-term priorities for service development. A complete review of the techniques that can be used by quality improvement groups is outside the scope of this chapter, but guidance is readily available (Oakland, 1993), (Lawrence and Schofield, 1993).

The group may use the techniques of clinical audit to collect information about care, identify particular aspects for improvement, recommend changes, and collect data once again. Simple techniques to encourage improvement may include the use of reminders and patient records, or structured records, or educational events for the team. Clinical audit has a central role to play. The use of systematically developed audit criteria can ensure that the team is improving its care according to the best available research evidence (Baker and Fraser, 1995). When combined with objective methods of data collection to check compliance with the criteria and appropriate strategies for changing performance when necessary, audit can lead to changes in performance which have an important impact on patient outcomes.

Co-operation and communication are the fundamental requirements for introducing many of these approaches (case study 5.2). Leadership can be the deciding factor in ensuring that a team works effectively and that communication is taking place. In many multi-partner practices there is no recognizable leadership, with the result that partners compete with each other. In others, however, leaders have been appointed to deal with specific issues or natural leaders have been accepted. An effective leader is someone who ensures that all members of the team are enabled to participate and that they feel involved and taken seriously. Ineffective leadership will lead to some members of the team becoming disenchanted and failing to pull their weight.

Team building through workshops or facilitation is one approach to enable teams to work together more effectively. There is a limited amount of evidence to show that facilitation can help (Hearnshaw, Baker and Robertson, 1994). Teams that are having problems may be well advised to seek the support of the local health authority or clinical audit group in gaining access to team building activities. However,

Quality example
The role of co-operation and communication

Teams
Teams need:
• leaders
• to be built

alone this may be insufficient unless it is coupled with an arrangement for continued effective leadership within the team.

CONTINUOUS MONITORING AND IMPROVEMENT

Genuine quality improvement will only be attained if a permanent system is in place to appraise and manage the quality of care. A critical component of such a quality system is the mechanism used to monitor the success of efforts to improve. The model in Figure 5.1 indicates that each quality group reports back on a regular basis. It may be that management needs to respond to recommendations from the group to modify the organization of services or to make new investments in facilities or staff. Management must also ascertain the reasons for failure of quality improvement, should that occur. The annual report of the team should include an overview of the quality system, detailing the problems in care that have been identified, those that were selected as priorities in the past year, progress that has been made in resolving these problems, and the problems that will be addressed in the next year. In this way, quality will become a continuing team management responsibility, rather than an afterthought subject to the whim of individual team members.

Over a period of time, new problems will inevitably arise. New policies will be identified by the health service, and new approaches to disease prevention and management will become available. The provision of quality care to elderly patients therefore requires a dynamic system that can not only respond to issues as they are brought to notice, but also plan ahead, anticipating future developments and exploring innovations in care.

This chapter has described a plan for quality improvement that can be used by primary health care teams. The details will vary to accommodate the different patterns of primary health care teams, but the principles are generally applicable. The combination of commitment, a continuing systematic approach and effective teamwork can correct many of the preventable instances of deficient care. Teams should now consider building on their experiences of clinical audit and improved team management to introduce quality improvement systems that improve the quality of primary health care for elderly people.

REFERENCES

Baker, R. (1996) Characteristics of patients, practices and general practitioners related to levels of patients' satisfaction with consultations. *British Journal of General Practice*, 46.

Baker, R. and Fraser, R.C. (1995) The development of review criteria linking guidelines and quality assessment. *British Medical Journal*, **311**, 370–3.

Baker, R., French, D., Lakhani, M. and Khunti, K. (1994) *Comments, Suggestions and Complaints*. Audit Protocol PC5. Eli Lilly National Clinical Audit Centre, Department of General Practice, University of Leicester, Leicester.

Baker, R. and Streatfield, J. (1995) What type of general practice do patients prefer? Exploration of practice characteristics influencing patient satisfaction. *British Journal of General Practice*, **45**, 654–9.

Baker, R., Sorrie, R., Reddish, S. *et al.* (1995) The facilitation of multiprofessional clinical audit in primary health care teams – from audit to quality assurance. *Journal of Interprofessional Care*, **9**, 237–44.

Baker, R., Whitfield, M. (1992) Measuring patient satisfaction: a test of construct validity. Quality in Health Care, **1**, 104–9.

Davis, D.A., Thomson, M.A., Oxman, A.D. and Haynes, R.B. (1995) Changing physician performance. A systematic review of the effect of continuing medical education strategies. *Journal of the American Medical Association*, **274**, 700–705.

Ebrahim, S. (1996) Caring for older people. Ethnic elders. *British Medical Journal*, **313**, 610–3.

Eccles, M., Clapp, Z. and Grimshaw, J. *et al.* (1996) North of England evidence based guidelines development project: methods of guideline development. *British Medical Journal*, **312**, 760–2.

Forbes, A. (1996) Caring for older people. Loneliness. *British Medical Journal*, **313**, 352–4.

Fotherby, M.D., Harper, G.D. and Potter, J.F. (1992) General Practitioners' management of hypertension in elderly patients. *British Medical Journal*, **305**, 750–2.

Gill, P., Dowell, A.C., Neal R.D. *et al.* (1996) Evidence based general practice: a retrospective study of interventions in one training practice. *British Medical Journal*, **312**, 819–21.

Grimshaw, J.M. and Russell, I.T. (1994) Achieving health gain through clinical guidelines II: ensuring guidelines change medical practice. *Quality in Health Care*, **3**, 45–52.

Grol, R. (1992) Implementing guidelines in general practice care. *Quality in Health Care*, **1**, 184–91.

Hearnshaw, H.M. (1993) The audit cycle managed by the primary care team. *Audit Trends*, **3**, 89–93.

Hearnshaw, H.M., Baker, R. and Robertson, N. (1994) Multidisciplinary audit in primary healthcare teams: facilitation by audit support staff. *Quality in Health Care*, **3**, 164–8.

Hicks, N.R. and Baker, I.A. (1991) General practitioners' opinions of health services available to their patients. *British Medical Journal*, **302**, 991–3.

Institute of Medicine (1992) *Guidelines for Clinical Practice. From development to use* (eds MJ Field and KN Lohr), Washington, DC: National Academy Press.

Jachuck, S.J. and Mulcaahy, J.R. (1987) Minimum data set necessary to promote the care of the elderly in general practice. *Journal of the Royal College of General Practitioners*, **37**, 207–9.

Jarman, B. (1985) Underprivileged areas, in *The Medical Annual 1985* (ed. DJP Gray), Wright, Bristol.

Krueger, R.A. (1988) *Focus Groups. A practical guide for applied research*. Newbury Park, California: Sage Publications Inc.

Lawrence, M. and Schofield, T. (1993) *Medical Audit in Primary Health Care*, Oxford University Press, Oxford.

Murray, S.A., Tapson, J., Turnball, L. *et al.* (1994). Listening to local voices: adapting rapid appraisal to access health and social needs in general practice. *British Medical Journal*, **308**, 698–700.

MacDonald, A.J.D. (1986) Do general practitioners 'miss' depression in elderly patients? *British Medical Journal*, **292**, 1365–7.

NHS Executive (1996). *Clinical Guidelines. Using clinical guidelines to improve patient care within the NHS*, London: Department of Health.

Oakland, J.S. (1993) *Total Quality Management*. Second edition. Butterworth-Heinemann Ltd, Oxford.

Philp, I. and Young, J. (1988). Audit of support given to lay carers of the demented elderly by a primary care team. *Journal of the Royal College of General Practitioners*, **38**, 153–5.

Pringle, M., Bradley, C.P., Carmichael, C.M., *et al.*, (1995) *Significant event auditing. A study of the feasibility and potential of case-based auditing in primary medical care*. Occasional paper 70. London: Royal College of General Practitioners.

Robertson, N., Baker, R. and Hearnshaw, H. (1996). Changing the clinical behaviour of doctors – a psychological framework. *Quality in Health Care*, **5**, 51–4.

Royal College of General Practitioners (1995) *The development and implementation of clinical guidelines. Report from practice 26*, London: Royal College of General Practitioners.

Sackett, D.L. and Rosenberg, W.M.C. (1995) The need for evidence-based medicine. *Journal of the Royal Society of Medicine*, **88**, 620–4.

Stern, M.C. and Jagger, C., Clark, E.M. *et al.* (1993) Residential care for elderly people: a decade of change. *British Medical Journal*, **306**, 827–30.

Sinclair, A.J. and Barnett, A.A. (1993). Special needs of elderly diabetic patients. *British Medical Journal*, **306**, 1142–3.

Teale, C. (1996) Caring for older people. Money problems and financial help. *British Medical Journal*, **313**, 288–90.

Vetter, N.J., Lewis, P.A. and Llewellyn, L. (1992) Supporting elderly dependent people at home. *British Medical Journal*, **304**, 1290–2.

Williams, E.I. and Fitton, F. (1991) Survey of carers of elderly patients discharged from hospital. *British Journal of General Practice*, **41**, 105–8.

Community care 6

David Challis and Karen Traske

EDITORS' INTRODUCTION

This chapter widens our consideration of the sectors of care
by looking at 'community care'. Changes are occurring in
systems of care for elderly people in many countries, usually
ascribed to the pressures of ageing populations and the costs
of care. This chapter analyses the development of community
care in the UK and how high quality community care can be
achieved, drawing on international experience.

This chapter is made up of four main parts. Initially the
reader is introduced to the underlying global trends in community care and what is driving these major changes. This is
followed by a description of the origins and nature of the new
community care policy in the UK. This tells how a policy came
out and was brought to life. Next, the authors use the UK
example to examine in detail the key issues in delivering high
quality community care. The issues include funding, needs
assessment, home care, care management and the health/
social care interface. Each of these is discussed in detail by
analysing the main goal, what can be achieved and the un-
solved challenges. The chapter ends by speculating about
future developments with the underlying theme of improving
interfaces – between secondary care and community care,
across organizational boundaries in general, and with other
areas such as housing policy.

After reading this chapter, you will have a comprehensive
picture of all aspects of community care. The chapter has a
strong political flavour in that it narrates how major policy
develops. Indeed this chapter will connect directly to the
experience of many readers yet the authors combine this with
down to earth advice, drawing on their research experience
and knowledge of other international developments.

Key topics
- International trends
- UK community care policy
- Implementation issues
- Looking forward

Quality Care for Elderly People. Edited by Peter P. Mayer, Edward J.
Dickinson and Martin Sandler. Published in 1997 by Chapman & Hall,
London. ISBN 0 412 61830 3

INTERNATIONAL TRENDS

Changes are occurring in systems of care for elderly people in many countries, and many of these must be ascribed to the pressures of an ageing population. At the same time, it is commonly believed that previous patterns of care for frail elderly people, which relied substantially upon institutional care, are no longer tenable. In a comparative study of changes in the care systems for elderly people in three European countries, The Netherlands, Sweden and the UK, Kraan *et al.* (1991) identified four common features:

- a move from standardized to flexible services
- a move from implicit to explicit interaction with informal care
- a move from bureaucratic centralism to regulated pluralism
- a move from separate to integrated social and economic criteria.

If we simplify these and look at patterns of change at the service level, it is possible to observe three interdependent forms of change: first, reduced reliance upon institutional patterns of provision; second, the enhancement of home-based care; and third, the development of improved systems of co-ordination at the patient or client level through the mechanism of case or care management. This pattern of changes in community care in different countries has been typified as providing a convergence, reflecting similar goals and policies, despite apparently varied organizational and funding structures (Challis, Davies and Traske, 1994a). Factors influencing this pattern of change include concerns about poor targeting and assessment, inappropriate placement of elderly people, the need to support carers and families, and the projected rising costs of institutional care.

Similar issues have been cited in Sweden (Johansson and Thorslund, 1991), The Netherlands (Tunissen and Knapen, 1991), France (Guillemard and Frossard, 1993), Germany (Dieck, 1993), Israel (Morginstin and Shamai, 1988), Australia (Ozanne, 1990), Japan (Golden Plan, 1990) and Canada (Ministries of Health, Community and Social Services, and Citizenship, 1993). Despite the similarity of the policy changes, it is important to note the critical contextual differences. First, although most countries intend to place less reliance upon institutional long-term care than hitherto in

Main strategic themes
- Flexibility
- Role of lay care
- Regulated 'pluralism'
- Integrated systems

Main service themes
- Less institutional care
- Better home care
- Improved care co-ordination

Drivers for change
- Poor targeting
- Inappropriate care
- Concern for carers
- Costs of care

the care of elderly people, a marginal shift in the proportion of those in nursing home care in The Netherlands, where 11% of elderly people are in nursing homes, is markedly different to the shift in the UK, where only some 5% of elderly people are in institutional care.

Second, divisions within service systems will vary according to historical usage in different countries. The divide between health and social care created in the UK is different to the system in Canada, where more home care is provided by the health service, or in Sweden where separation of responsibilities is not between health and social care but between acute and long-term care (Thorslund and Parker, 1994).

UK COMMUNITY CARE POLICY

Background and origins

The current structure of services for elderly people reflects the restructuring of the early 1970s. In 1970, following the Seebohm Report (Cmnd 3703), the Local Authority Social Services Act was passed. This created social services departments which took on responsibility for certain services that had previously been under local authority health departments (social workers, home helps, meals services and day centres).

In 1974, health services were reorganized to create district health authorities. Local authority health care provision such as community nursing was transferred to the district health authorities, and hospital social work was transferred to the social services departments.

Since the White Paper *Health and Welfare: the Development of Community Care* (Cmnd 1973) in 1963, community care for elderly people has been a long-standing policy objective. The creation of the local authority social services departments was expected to lead to improved services for elderly people and to extend community care provision. These expectations were not, however, fulfilled. For example, although the proportion of total social services department expenditure on elderly people increased from 38.1% to 45% between 1973 and 1979, the percentage allocated to community services remained the same and continued thus into the mid-1980s (Parker, 1990). Hence, overall expenditure increased due to the growing number of elderly people in the population, but there was no shift in the way in which resources were allocated. Moreover, studies suggested that community care was not sufficient or comprehensive enough to act as a substitute for institutional care (Goldberg and Connelly, 1982; Johnson et al., 1983; Sinclair et al., 1990).

In their review of social care research Goldberg and Connelly (1982) conclude:

> Numerous local enquiries have repeatedly thrown up similar issues in many different spheres of social care; the mismatch between needs and resources, the inadequacy of appropriate initial assessment and the lack of monitoring and review procedures.

A phase of conflicting policy
- Easy access to funding for institutional care (national social security)
- Limited funds for home care (local social services)

During the 1980s the long-standing official policy of community care, in which the social services were expected to play a major part, was thwarted by the unforseen consequences of financial restraint. In the face of growing needs arising from an ageing population, the only major source of funding available for long-term care was through the social security system. This was allocated purely according to financial need, and enabled many elderly people to enter private and voluntary residential and nursing homes. Conversely, the funds available for social services departments and health authorities to develop home-based care were limited as part of an overall policy to restrain public spending. A serious distortion in policy thus arose, so that between 1980 and 1989 the expenditure on places in residential and nursing provision in the non-statutory sector rose from £10 million to £1000 million (Cm 849).

An influential report by the Audit Commission (1986) examined the pattern of development of community care and noted in particular the organizational fragmentation and confusion of service systems, the mismatch of resources to needs, and the perverse incentives towards the growth of institutional care created by the system of funding. The ready availability of social security funds for institutional care provided little logical financial basis for agencies to invest in intensive home care services. In response, the Government appointed Sir Roy Griffiths as a special adviser to report on possible strategies for community care. His report, published in 1988, recommended a more consolidated and co-ordinated approach to the funding and management of care, placing responsibility for the allocation of funds, assessment of need and co-ordination of care with the local authority social serv-

---

An identified need for
- consolidation
- integration
- clarification
- co-ordination

ices department. To focus resources effectively for the most vulnerable, care management was recommended (Griffiths, 1988).

The new community care policy

The majority of these recommendations were accepted by the Government in its policy document *Caring for People*, published in 1989 (Cm 849), where six key objectives were identified for community care (Box 6.1). To achieve these objectives a number of structural and organizational changes were effected (Box 6.2). First, social services departments became the only source of public funding for the social care of elderly people, to eliminate perverse incentives. Second, the social services departments became the lead agency in assessing the needs of individuals, for deciding the mix of services that would best suit those needs, and monitoring and reviewing the quality of care provided. In future, placement in residential and nursing homes was therefore to be on the basis of assessed need rather than financial eligibility.

A mixed economy of care – public, private and voluntary – was expected to develop. The social services department was

---

The resultant policy
- Clear objectives
- New funding structure
- Single lead agency
- Provision based on need

Policy objectives
- Promotion of home care
- Support for carers
- Needs assessment and care management
- Mixed economy
- Clear responsibilities
- Better value for money

Box 6.1   UK community care policy objectives

- To promote the development of domiciliary, day and respite services to enable people to live in their own homes wherever feasible and sensible.
- To ensure that service providers make practical support for carers a high priority.
- To make proper assessment of need and good case management the cornerstone of high quality care.
- To promote the development of a flourishing independent sector alongside good quality public services.
- To clarify the responsibilities of agencies and so make it easier to hold them to account for their performance.
- To secure better value for taxpayers' money by introducing a new funding structure for social care.

(Source: Cm 849 (1989) Paragraph 1.11.)

Box 6.2   UK community care policy: structural and organizational changes

- Integration of funding. A new funding structure placing responsibility for the financial support of those who enter residential care with the local authority through its social services department, which would have to assess their need for such a placement. The social security funds spent on residential care were to be transferred to the local authorities.
- Assessment and co-ordination of care. Local authority social service departments to be responsible, in collaboration with medical, nursing and other interests, for assessing individual need, designing care arrangements and securing their delivery within available resources. Assessment would be undertaken both for people seeking day and domiciliary care services and for those seeking admission to publicly funded residential and nursing home care. These activities would include the appointment of care managers for individuals such as vulnerable elderly people when it was appropriate.
- Mixed economy of care. Local authorities will be expected to make maximum use of the independent sector in providing care services.
- Community care planning. Local authorities will produce and publish clear plans for the development of community care services in their areas, consistent with the plans of health authorities and other agencies.
- Inspection and registration. Local authorities must establish inspection and registration units which will monitor standards, both in their own residential accommodation and in the independent sector.

(Source: Cm 849 (1989) Paragraph 1.12.)

expected to move from the role of monopoly provider to that of the 'enabling authority' which, through purchasing, contracting and planning, would be both a provider of services and a creator of a market of care, taking account of local needs and demands. As lead agency, social services departments were each expected to produce integrated community care plans and also to arrange for the registration and inspection of all residential and nursing homes.

KEY ISSUES IN THE DEVELOPMENT OF COMMUNITY CARE

The effective implementation of this policy in practice will depend upon several factors, both explicit and implicit (Box 6.2). These are: funding arrangements, needs assessment, home-based care, care management and the interface between health and social care.

Funding arrangements

In order to remove the perverse incentive which had made funding available for unassessed placements in residential and nursing home care, but not for own home-based care, public funding was consolidated in the hands of the social services department. This involved bringing together the social security monies with the base budget of the social services department. However, this consolidation was far from complete.

First, a substantial amount of long-term institutional expenditure has traditionally been made by health authorities in the form of continuing care beds, but the number of these has been reduced and there has been no transfer of this element to social services, which has thus diminished the amount of resources used for long-term care. Second, despite the objective that all future publicly funded entrants to residential and nursing homes would be assessed, it is still feasible for people to amass combinations of benefits which permit them to bypass the assessment system using social security funds (Wistow and Henwood, 1994). A third concern about funding, likely to be of increasing importance as charging policies for services increase, is that of the potential cost of long-term care for broader family units. Although estimates from both the USA and the UK suggest that the market for private insurance for long-term care is restricted, there is likely to be room for further consideration of the role of insurance in such areas as asset protection (Challis, Davies and Traske, 1994b).

There has been debate both about the size of the allocation of funds to make the policy feasible, and also the means

Main goal
- Remove perverse incentives

Key issues
- Funding
- Needs assessment
- Home care
- Care management
- Health–social care interface

by which those funds are distributed between different local authorities. Approaches that distributed resources on the basis of current numbers of residential and nursing home beds have been seen as disadvantaging urban areas, and distribution that reflected population levels of older people in the second year of the policy have been seen as disadvantaging other areas. The process of allocating central funding equitably to local needs is likely to be a continuing concern.

Needs assessment

Assessment of need and good care management were identified as the cornerstone of high quality care in the new community care arrangements, as shown in Box 6.1 (Cm 849). Although assessment is mandatory, the form that assessment takes is not at all prescribed. Early Department of Health monitoring has suggested that assessments of elderly people tend to be excessively variable in form, too frequently monodisciplinary in nature and insufficiently problem-focused (Department of Health, 1993). The contribution of health care staff to assessment, particularly the critical assessments involving decisions about placement of elderly people in institutional care, is dependent upon local negotiation. Interestingly, there is no prescribed role for secondary health care services such as geriatrics and psychogeriatrics in this process, which might make comprehensive multidisciplinary assessment possible. Studies suggest that geriatric screening may detect previously unrecognized disease and/or reduce the probability of inappropriate admission to institutional care (Brocklehurst, Carty and Leeming, 1978; Rafferty, Smith and Williamson, 1987; Kalra and Foster, 1989; Stuck et al., 1993; Peet et al., 1994).

The Australian Aged Care Reforms provide an interesting contrast. Faced with the dramatic growth in nursing home care, comprehensive assessment prior to placement became mandatory. Geriatric assessment teams were developed to screen all publicly funded admissions to residential and nursing home care. Following implementation, between 1986 and 1990, the number of nursing home beds per 1000 aged over 70 decreased by 15%. Of 2006 cases referred for nursing home care assessment in the state of Victoria, only 55% were thus placed, the remainder being distributed between residential homes, acute treatment and home care (Otis, 1992). Another study suggests a 38% diversion rate

---

Main goal
- Provision based on need

Challenges
- Variation in methods
- Involving disciplines
- Health and social care collaboration
- Using specialized health care expertise

Quality example
- In Australia, special assessment teams screen potential long-term care residents

following comprehensive assessment (Quartararo and O'Neill, 1990). It is interesting to speculate whether such a role could be developed in the UK to evaluate placement decisions.

Home-based care

Home help and community nursing have tended to be the most frequently used services, and much of the available evidence suggests that these are highly valued by elderly people (Sinclair *et al.*, 1990). During the 1980s there was a general trend towards encouraging greater targeting of use, particularly of home help services, so as to permit greater amounts of care to be provided for the most vulnerable elderly people. Criticisms of services focused upon this lack of intensity, failure to provide adequate support to carers and insufficiently flexible responses (Goldberg and Connelly, 1982; Sinclair *et al.*, 1990). In response to this the Social Services Inspectorate increased the intensity of home care provision (Social Services Inspectorate, 1987), and the development of specialized forms of enhanced home care (both to permit earlier hospital discharge and to provide home-based long-term care).

A study that provided augmented home care to discharge elderly people from acute hospital beds proved unsuccessful due to the imbalance between the small amount of service available in relation to the degree of need of the patients (Victor and Vetter, 1988). The importance of focused and intensive support was confirmed in a second study, which provided specialized support for patients over the age of 75 being discharged from hospital. Specially employed care assistants provided help for up to 12 hours per week for two weeks after discharge. They undertook a wide range of tasks, personal and household care, as well as stimulation and encouragement to increase activity levels. The number of days spent in hospital by those receiving the service was reduced compared with those in a control population (Townsend *et al.*, 1988).

Innovations have also taken place in long-term care. One study of intensive home nursing and augmented home care provided up to 21 hours per week of home help, and offered an alternative to long-stay hospital care. Although it was a small study with few outcome data, its package of care appeared to be a less costly alternative for mentally intact but physically disabled elderly people (Gibbins *et al.*, 1982).

Challenges
- Lack of intensive home care
- Lack of specialized home care

Quality example
- Augmented home care to support hospital discharge

Quality examples
- Augmented home care to replace long-term care
- Flexible respite care

Other interventions have included a specialized unit offering respite, evening and occasional residential care for mentally infirm elderly people and their carers. Although costly, this appeared to reduce admissions to long-stay hospital care (Donaldson and Gregson, 1989).

The conclusion that appears to emerge from numerous studies of home-based care is that simply expanding the level and extent of provision is a necessary, but not sufficient, condition for it to substitute for institutional care (Davies *et al.*, 1990; Sinclair *et al.*, 1990; Jamieson, 1991). In order to supply the necessary focusing of effort, development of service at the margin and co-ordination of care, care management has a role to play.

> **Practice point**
> To be successful, home care:
> • must be provided at appropriate levels
> • must be focused

Care management

> **Main goal**
> • Individualized, flexible and co-ordinated packages of care
>
> **Practice point**
> Key elements of care management:
> • cost framework
> • control of resources
> • flexibility

Part of the strategy of community-based care policies in many countries has been described in The Netherlands as 'downward substitution'. Co-ordination of care for vulnerable individuals by care managers is seen as one approach to offering home care of a sufficiently comprehensive kind to act as an alternative to institutional care. A major series of evaluations in intensive care management in the long-term care of elderly people has been undertaken at the Personal Social Services Research Unit [PSSRU] at the University of Kent. These have involved the exploration of a model of care management that devolved control of resources within an overall cost framework to individual care managers, so that they could respond more flexibly to needs. The model was examined with deliberate and planned variation in settings and target groups, within an overall focus on very vulnerable elderly people

Table 6.1   PSSRU care management studies: settings and target groups*

Study	Setting	Target population
Kent Community Care Project	Social care/SSD care+	Residential
Gateshead Community Care Scheme	Social care/SSD care+	Residential
Gateshead Health and Social Care	SSD/primary care Hospital/residential/nursing home care	
Darlington Community Care Project	Geriatric long-stay multidisciplinary team care/SSD	Hospital

*Source: Challis and Davies, 1986; Challis *et al.*, 1988, 1990, 1991a, 1991b, 1995.

(Table 6.1). The target groups ranged from elderly people on the margin of admission to residential care homes, to those requiring long-stay hospital care. Care managers were located in social services departments, as members of a single discipline team, in primary health care, and in secondary health care multidisciplinary teams such as geriatric medicine.

These studies indicated that care managers with greater budgetary flexibility were able to respond more effectively. The care provided was more individually varied, and control of a budget meant that assessments became more wide-ranging and problem-focused. Consequently, a number of problems often associated with the breakdown of community care, such as severe stress on carers, confusional states, and risk of falling, were more effectively managed at home than in the comparison groups.

As shown in Box 6.3, the need for institutional care for vulnerable elderly people was reduced. The level of well-being of elderly people and their carers was usually significantly improved, and this was achieved at no greater, and sometimes less, cost to the social and health services and society as a whole. These studies indicate that positive outcomes and diversion from institutional care are most likely to occur when the service is carefully targeted on vulnerable

---

Practice point
Care management leads to:
- flexible care packages
- problem orientation
- improved outcomes
- same or reduced cost

Box 6.3   PSSRU care management studies: main findings

Compared with the usual patterns of service provision, elderly people receiving intensive care management services:

- received a wider and more intensive range of home care services
- were able to remain in their own homes for longer
- were less likely to enter institutional long-term care
- experienced improved quality of life, as did their carers
- had similar or lower levels of health and social services costs

(Source: Challis and Davies, 1986; Challis *et al.*, 1988, 1990, 1991b, 1995)

individuals at risk of institutional care, albeit with relatively modest cost savings (Challis and Davies, 1986; Kemper, 1988; Challis *et al.*, 1990, 1991a, 1991b, 1995).

In the UK community care reforms, it is possible to interpret the Department of Health guidance (SSI/SWSG, 1991) as implying that care management principles be applied to all recipients of community care. This raises the problem of how to spread the overhead costs of care management across cases for whom there is little or no probability of diversion from institutional care, and who may be relatively low consumers of domiciliary services (Department of Health, 1994). Since the available research evidence indicates the benefits of care management are likely to be greatest with restricted target groups, a more precise definition is required. One solution is to discriminate between, on the one hand, 'intensive care management', meaning the provision of designated care managers for those with severe, complex and potentially volatile needs, and, on the other, a more effective system of organizational procedures for assessment, care plans and reviews for a wider range of service recipients (Challis, 1994).

Inevitably, the precise boundary between intensive care management and organizational process will be determined not only by evidence of effectiveness, policy definition and need, but also by resource factors such as the availability of trained staff. Nonetheless, this targeting question is likely to prove central to the introduction of care management in social care, since it is critical to the capacity to provide sufficiently comprehensive home-based care as a real alternative to institutional care. A helpful analogy would be to place intensive care management in the same relationship to mainstream domiciliary care services as secondary health care services are to GPs.

One way to achieve a more focused approach to intensive care management might be to develop further structural linkages with health care services. Although general practice is often seen as a possible setting for care management, it may well be the case that the main benefits of general practice would be for case-finding rather than the provision of continuing care. For example, the role of GPs in screening elderly people over the age of 75 may identify unmet social care needs, and would also provide access to members of the primary health care team for their contributions to assessment and home support. Conversely, the number of elderly

---

Practice point
Care management needs:
- targeting
- concentration of effort
- associated care systems for other clients

people requiring intensive care management would be likely to be relatively small on any one GP's list, and there may be a case for locating intensive care management in secondary health care settings, such as geriatric services (Challis *et al.*, 1991a, 1991b, 1995), or a community mental health team for elderly people (Murphy and Challis, 1993).

The Australian experience provides an interesting comparison. The development of geriatric assessment teams has already been discussed as a means of avoiding misplacement of elderly people in institutional care. A further, but related, element of the community care changes in that country has been the development of case management as an alternative to institutional care. In the state of Victoria, referrals to the Community Options Projects, which were to provide case management, were channelled through the geriatric assessment teams and, in two projects, case management was physically located within the geriatric assessment team (Kendig *et al.*, 1992). This provided a link between multidisciplinary assessment at the point of potential placement and the immediate availability of alternative diversionary services.

The mid-term review of the Australian Aged Care Policy (Department of Community Services and Health 1991) indicated that there was further scope for linking case management with geriatric assessment teams. A similar conclusion emerged in the evaluation of the Community Options Programme (Department of Health, Housing and Community Services, 1992), which indicated that closer links between geriatric assessment teams and case managers were beneficial in managing problems of mobility, incontinence and dementia. Importantly, it appeared that such links had also enabled geriatric assessment teams to become more integrated into the mainstream community care network.

The Australian experience is an interesting one for the UK, with its network of widely developed geriatric services. However, whereas in Australia there is a specifically defined role for geriatric assessment services in community care, namely assessment and screening, no such formal role exists in the UK, and such arrangements are entirely dependent upon local negotiation. In Australia it has been suggested that by linking geriatric assessment and case management 'the clinical and diagnostic skills of assessment teams could be more widely used by [case management] projects in their

> **Quality example**
> Community options projects – linking clinical skills to care management

assessment and care planning functions' (Department of Health, Housing and Community Services, 1992, p. 97). It would seem that the relationship between community care, geriatric medicine and other secondary health care services is one that offers opportunities for further worthwhile experimentation.

The interface between health and social care

The current separation of health and social care in the UK owes much to the pattern of organizational change in the early 1970s described at the beginning of this chapter. Since that time, the boundary of that separation, born more of organizational convenience than logical response to patient need, has become more unclear. As the policies for re-focusing home care services to meet personal care needs have developed, and the health service has retreated from the provision of continuing care, the boundary poses not just planning problems between the two main agencies but also real dilemmas for patients and their families regarding payment for care that might once have been free under the health service. The development of community care has made this problem both more acute and more visible.

Even the most well-meaning attempts to discriminate between health and social care responsibilities for particular tasks illustrate the problem graphically by their inability to do so. For example, of the 20 tasks relevant to elderly people that are used to illustrate the division of social and health care responsibilities in the managers' guide to care management and assessment (Social Services Inspectorate and Social Work Services Group, 1991), only six were allocated to social care, five to health care and nine could be performed by either agency. Such a search for precise discrimination by task may ultimately prove unfeasible, and alternative approaches may be more helpful. As Ebrahim argues, the specialty of health care for the elderly is founded 'on the principle of comprehensiveness of care – be it social or medical – and . . . that, for effective management of patients . . . blurring the boundaries of health and social care is the **mechanism** by which seamless care is achieved' (Ebrahim, 1994, p. 298). In many ways, what is emerging is a separation between health and social care that is actually a division of responsibility between acute and chronic care but without the transfer of staff and resources necessary to make such an arrangement fully effective.

Main goal
• Seamless care

Challenges
• What is 'social'?
• What is 'health'?
• Who pays?

In Sweden, the division of health and social care posed similar problems, and in 1992 services for elderly and disabled people were reorganized, with the municipalities, which were already responsible for housing and social welfare services, also taking the responsibility for long-term medical care. The administration of nursing homes and own home medical care was also transferred to the municipalities, which also became financially responsible for patients in acute hospitals once treatment was completed, thereby addressing the issue of bed-blocking (Thorslund and Parker, 1994). These changes are interesting because they address the problem of the health and social care divide by creating an acute and chronic care separation, with the whole range of necessary staff and resources transferred to effect that process. Observing the effects of these changes will be of interest to many, given the problematic separation of health and social care in other countries.

An alternative organizational scenario in the UK is posed by the arrangements in Northern Ireland. There, integrated health and social service boards are responsible for the provision of both health and social care. A mix of the staff necessary to provide long-term care is available within integrated provider unit trusts, thus avoiding the disincentives that make it difficult to use nursing staff as care managers in the rest of the UK. The progress of community care reforms in Northern Ireland and the extent to which the health and social service boards, possessing integrated budgets, are able to bridge the health and social care divide is also likely to be of continuing interest.

LOOKING FORWARD

Clearly the development of a new community care policy in the UK is at an early stage, and any pronouncement on its effectiveness would be, to say the least, premature. However, we have attempted to identify a number of areas of critical importance which may need to be addressed if the desired policy goals and improved home-based care are to be achieved for elderly people. As in policy changes in many other countries, assessment is the starting point for long-term care arrangements. We have discussed some of the possible opportunities for linking geriatric and other secondary care services more closely with community-based care to improve the quality of assessment and placement

> **Quality example**
> In Sweden, health services are only responsible for acute care

> **Quality example**
> In Northern Ireland, health and social service boards are integrated

> **Nurturing development**
> • Linking specialized hospital services and community care
> • Resolving boundary issues
> • Interface with housing

decisions, with particular reference to the experience in Australia.

The policy of 'downward substitution' is likely to depend on the success of the development of intensive care management (Challis, 1994). However, it would seem at present that, as in the previous development of home care services, care management is in danger of being more thinly spread and less intensive than is necessary (Department of Health, 1994). One interesting opportunity that could contribute to resolving this problem would be closer links between intensive care management and geriatric and other secondary health care services (Challis *et al.*, 1995).

There remain, however, organizational barriers to some of the most clinically relevant approaches to the provision of long-term care, often arising from the boundaries between health and social care. Whether current boundaries can be made to work through the enlightened application of joint purchasing (Audit Commission, 1992), or whether further organizational changes towards the models operating in Northern Ireland or Sweden will prove necessary, remains an open question.

A final consideration must be that effective community care is not dependent on the efforts of health and social care alone, but also on the provision of suitable and adequate housing. There are examples of care management schemes that have failed precisely because of this lack. It is probable that our conception of community care is likely to become more subtle over time, as the development of more finely differentiated forms of supported housing breaks down the current binary distinction between institutional and community care (Challis *et al.*, 1994b).

REFERENCES

Audit Commission (1986) *Making a Reality of Community Care*, HMSO, London.

Audit Commission (1992) *Community Care: Managing the Cascade of Change*, HMSO, London.

Brocklehurst, J.C., Carty, M.H. and Leeming, J.T. (1978) Care of the elderly: medical screening of old people accepted for residential care. *Lancet*, **ii**, 141–2.

Challis, D. (1994) Care Management: Factors Influencing its Development in the Implementation of Community Care, *Implementing Caring for People*, Department of Health, London.

Challis, D. and Davies, B. (1986) *Case Management in Community Care*, Gower, Aldershot.

Challis, D., Davies, B. and Traske, K. (1994a) Community care: promise, ambition and imperative – an international agenda, in *Community Care: New Agendas and Challenges from the UK and Overseas* (eds D. Challis, B. Davies and K. Traske), Arena, Aldershot.

Challis, D., Davies, B. and Traske, K. (1994b) Community care: immediate concerns and long-term perspectives, in *Community Care: New Agendas and Challenges from the UK and Overseas* (eds D. Challis, B. Davies and K. Traske), Arena, Aldershot.

Challis, D., Chessum, R., Chesterman, J. *et al.* (1988) Community Care for the frail elderly: an urban experiment. *British Journal of Social Work*, **18**(Supplement), 43–54.

Challis, D., Chessum, R., Chesterman, J. *et al.* (1990) *Case Management in Social and Health Care*, Personal Social Services Research Unit, University of Kent at Canterbury, Kent.

Challis, D., Darton, R., Johnson, L. *et al.* (1991a) An evaluation of an alternative to long-stay hospital care for frail elderly patients: Part I The model of care. *Age and Ageing*, **20**, 236–44.

Challis, D., Darton, R., Johnson, L. *et al.* (1991b) An evaluation of an alternative to long-stay hospital care for the frail elderly: Part II Costs and outcomes. *Age and Ageing*, **20**, 245–54.

Challis, D., Darton, R., Johnson, L. *et al.* (1995) *Care Management and Health Care of Older People: The Darlington Community Care Project*, Arena, Aldershot.

Cm 849 (1989) *Caring for People: Community Care in the Next Decade and Beyond*, HMSO, London.

Cmnd 1973 (1963) *Health and Welfare: The Development of Community Care*, HMSO, London.

Cmnd 3703 (1968) *Report of the Committee on Local Authority and Allied Personal Social Services*, HMSO, London.

Davies, B., Bebbington, A., Charnley, H. *et al.* (1990) *Resources, Needs and Outcomes in Community Care*, Gower, Aldershot.

Department of Community Services and Health (1991) *Aged Care Reform Strategy: Mid-Term Review 1990–91. Report*, Australian Publishing Service, Canberra.

Department of Health (1993) *Monitoring and Development: Assessment Special Study*, Department of Health, London.

Department of Health (1994) *Monitoring and Development: Care Management Special Study*, Department of Health, London.

Department of Health, Housing and Community Services (1992) *It's Your Choice: National Evaluation of Community Options Projects*, Aged and Community Care Division, Department of Health, Housing and Community Services, Australian Government Publishing Service, Canberra.

Dieck, M. (1993) Risks and achievements in strengthening home care: the example of Germany, in *Better Care for Dependent*

People Living at Home (eds A. Evers and G. van der Zanden), Netherlands Institute of Gerontology, Bunnik.

Donaldson, C. and Gregson, B. (1989) Prolonging life at home: what is the cost? *Community Medicine*, **11**(3), 200–9.

Ebrahim, S. (1994) Community care: implications for health services for elderly people, in *Community Care: New Agendas and Challenges from the UK and Overseas* (eds D. Challis, B. Davies and K. Traske), Arena, Aldershot.

Gibbins, F.J., Lee, M., Davison, P. *et al.* (1982) Augmented home nursing as an alternative to hospital care for chronic elderly invalids. *British Medical Journal*, **284**, 330–3.

Goldberg, E.M. and Connelly, N. (1982) *The Effectiveness of Social Care for the Elderly: An Overview of Recent and Current Evaluative Research*, Heinemann Educational Books, London.

Golden Plan (1990) *Ten Year Strategy to Promote Health Care and Welfare for the Aged* (English translation), Ministry of Health and Welfare, Tokyo.

Griffiths, R. (1988) *Community Care: Agenda for Action*, HMSO, London.

Guillemard, A. and Frossard, M. (1993) Risks and achievements in strengthening home care: the case of France, in *Better Care for Dependent People Living at Home* (eds A. Evers and G. van der Zanden), Netherlands Institute of Gerontology, Bunnik.

Jamieson, A. (1991) *Home Care for Older People in Europe*, Oxford University Press, Oxford.

Johansson, L. and Thorslund, M. (1991) The national context of social innovation – Sweden, in *Care for the Elderly: Significant Innovations in Three European Countries* (eds R.J. Kraan, J. Baldock, B. Davies *et al.*), Campus/Westview, Boulder, Colorado.

Johnson, M., Challis, D., Power, M. and Wade, B. (eds) (1983) The realities and potential of community care in DHSS, in *Elderly People in the Community: Their Service Needs*, HMSO, London.

Kalra, L. and Foster, C. (1989) Assessment of applicants for sheltered housing. *Age and Ageing*, **18**, 271–4.

Kemper, P. (1988) The evaluation of the national long-term care demonstration: 10. Overview of findings. *Health Services Research*, **23**(1), 161–74.

Kendig, H., McVicar, G., Reynolds, A. and O'Brien, A. (1992) *Victorian Linkages Evaluation*, Department of Health, Housing and Community Services, Canberra.

Kraan, R., Baldock, J., Davies, B. *et al.* (eds) (1991) *Care for the Elderly: Significant Innovations in Three European Countries*, Campus/Westview, Boulder, Colorado.

Ministries of Health, Community and Social Services, and Citizenship (1993) *Partnerships in Long-Term Care: A New Way to Plan, Manage and Deliver Services and Community Support. A Policy Framework*, Ministries of Health, Community and Social Services and Citizenship, Toronto, Ontario.

Morginstin, B. and Shamai, N. (1988) Issues in planning long-term care insurance in Israel's social security system. *Social Security: Journal of Welfare and Social Security Studies* (English edition), **30**, 31–48.

Murphy, E. and Challis, D. (eds) (1993) The Lewisham Care Management Scheme for people with dementia, in *Mental Health and Aging*, WHO, Geneva.

Otis, N. (1992) *Identifying Care Alternatives for Older People: The Victorian Regional Geriatric Assessment Programme*, Lincoln Papers in Gerontology 13, Lincoln Gerontology Centre, La Trobe University, Melbourne.

Ozanne, E. (1990) Development of Australian health and social policy in relation to the aged and the emergence of home care services, in *Community Care Policy and Practice: New Directions in Australia* (eds A. Howe, E. Ozanne and C. Selby Smith), Public Sector Management Institute, Monash University, Victoria.

Parker, R. (1990) Elderly people and community care: the policy background, in *The Kaleidoscope of Care: A Review of Research on Welfare Provision for Elderly People* (eds I. Sinclair, R. Parker, D. Leat and J. Williams), HMSO, London.

Peet, S.M., Castleden, C.M., Potter, J.F. and Jagger, C. (1994) The outcome of a medical examination for applicants to Leicestershire home for older people. *Age and Ageing*, **23**, 65–8.

Quartararo, M. and O'Neill, T.J. (1990) Nursing home admissions: the effect of a multidisciplinary assessment team on the frequency of admission approvals. *Community Health Studies*, **14**, 441–9.

Rafferty, J., Smith, R.G. and Williamson, J. (1987) Medical assessment of elderly persons prior to a move to residential care: a review of seven years' experience in Edinburgh. *Age and Ageing*, **16**, 10–12.

Sinclair, I., Parker, R., Leat, D. and Williams, J. (eds) (1990) *The Kaleidoscope of Care: A Review of Research on Welfare Provision for Elderly People*, HMSO, London.

Social Services Inspectorate (1987) *From Home Help to Home Care: An Analysis of Policy Resourcing and Service Management*, SSI, London.

Social Services Inspectorate and Social Work Services Group (1991) *Care Management and Assessment: Managers Guide*, Social Services Inspectorate and Social Work Services Group, HMSO, London.

Stuck, A.E., Siu, A.L., Wieland, G.D. *et al.* (1993) Comprehensive geriatric assessment: a meta analysis of controlled trials. *Lancet*, **342**, 1032–6.

Thorslund, M. and Parker, M. (1994) Care of the elderly in the changing Swedish welfare state, in *Community Care: New Agendas and Challenges from the UK and Overseas* (eds D.J. Challis, B. Davies and K. Traske), Arena, Aldershot.

Townsend, J., Piper, M., Frank, A. *et al.* (1988) Reduction in hospital readmission stay of elderly patients by a community based hospital discharge scheme: a randomised controlled trial. *British Medical Journal*, **297**, 544–7.

Tunissen, C. and Knapen, M. (1991) The national context of social innovation – The Netherlands, in *Care for the Elderly: significant Innovations in Three European Countries* (eds R.J. Kraan, J. Baldock, B. Davies *et al.*), Campus/Westview, Boulder, Colorado.

Victor, C.R. and Vetter, N.J. (1988) Rearranging the deckchairs on the Titanic: Failure of an augmented home help scheme after discharge to reduced the length of stay in hospital. *Archives of Gerontology and Geriatrics*, **7**, 83–91.

Wistow, G. and Henwood, M. (1994) Wrong way home. *Health Service Journal*, **23 June**, 26–7.

The private sector 7

Philip Tormey and Terry Devenney

EDITORS' INTRODUCTION

This chapter is concerned with the most rapidly growing sector of care – the private sector. Although in the care of elderly people this sector is mainly concerned with the provision of residential and nursing home care, changes are likely to occur. Often the contribution of the private sector may be underestimated or undervalued. This chapter details what the private sector has to offer now and in the future.

This chapter is made up of seven main sections. The first three sections are concerned with the important and complex relationships of the private sector with: the public sector; the new community care legislation; and with regulations. These sections form a backdrop for the subsequent three sections by describing the reality of community care and how this is affecting the private sector. There is a useful debate about the role of regulation, with the conclusion that reform is needed. The next major section is devoted to quality initiatives in the private sector. There is consideration of the assessment of outcomes of care and processes of care, with examples of how to involve residents and available quality initiatives. This leads to consideration of the role of training, which highlights the NVQ and Investors in People schemes and the need to make training practical to be effective. A fascinating section on the diversification of care explains why there has not been a rapid growth of alternative approaches. This is illustrated with reference to domiciliary care, outreach services, respite care and care villages. Finally, current issues are examined with special emphasis on those that require rapid solutions – the range of services, funding, and regulation. These are used as a springboard to indulge in

Key topics
- Relationship with the public sector
- Impact of new legislation
- Role of regulation
- Quality activities
- Training
- Diversification of care
- Current issues

Quality Care for Elderly People. Edited by Peter P. Mayer, Edward J. Dickinson and Martin Sandler. Published in 1997 by Chapman & Hall, London. ISBN 0 412 61830 3

some crystal ball gazing in relation to future trends in the role of the private sector.

After reading this chapter, you will have a clear understanding of the boundaries and constraints within which the private sector acts and the many ways in which it has responded to improve the quality of care of elderly people. This should assist readers from other sectors in dealing effectively with colleagues in the private sector. In particular, there may be much to gain from harmonizing quality activities across the sectors of care.

RELATIONSHIP WITH THE PUBLIC SECTOR

Public sector controls
- Setting standards
- Regulation
- Client placement
- Major purchaser

The private sector operates under the direct or indirect control of the public sector, which also provides a large proportion of its funding. The public sector sets and monitors standards, acts as regulator, assesses and places clients and is the major purchaser of private sector services. Despite this symbiotic relationship, there is considerable misunderstanding between the two, arising from their differing goals and concerns. Long-term residential care is now dominated by the private sector. The move away from a public sector supply of beds has been assisted by the scaling down of local authority Part III homes and the rise in demand (Laing and Buisson, 1993). The growth was considerably boosted by the acknowledgement of the unacceptable standard of care in long-stay NHS wards, which could neither provide the homely atmosphere and flexibility of smaller units desired by residents, families and carers, nor the necessary expansion (Royal College of Nursing, 1987).

Myths about private long-term care
- Profit unacceptable
- Huge profits
- Lower care standards

The perception of those in the public sector that the supply of long-term care 'for profit' is unpalatable remains strong and can act as a brake on the development of public/private sector co-operation in planning and delivery of services. Allied to this is the myth that huge profits are being made at the expense of residents (Independent Health Care Association, 1992). Furthermore, there is an unsubstantiated assumption that the public and voluntary sectors have higher standards of care (Llewellyn, 1993). The unplanned growth of the private sector, funded largely by social security payments, has resulted in an unevenness in the geographical supply of beds and in the types of services on offer. It is against this background that the private sector contribution to the care of elderly people must be considered.

IMPACT OF COMMUNITY CARE LEGISLATION

The new community care legislation has had, and will continue to have, an enormous impact on the structure and operation of the private care sector. Funding of care services largely passed to local authorities with a consequent increase in importance of local authority social services departments for the private care sector.

However, the new community care policy incorporated two little-understood flaws. The first flawed assumption was that the 'perverse incentives' of unassessed benefit payments was the cause for the rapid growth of private residential care (Audit Commission, 1988a). An alternative view is that a large number of people accessed a level of care that they could not otherwise have had (Firth Committee, 1987).

The Griffiths Report (Griffiths, 1988) contained the second flawed assumption: that domiciliary care could replace residential care for the majority because it was:

- a 'right' or 'natural' preference of individuals
- 'better' than residential care
- generally cheaper.

Recent developments have indicated that there is limited user right of choice between domiciliary and residential care. Further, domiciliary care is not better if only minimum needs are met, and 24-hour care by trained nurses can have many benefits such as lower readmission rates to hospitals (Clark, 1992). Finally, there is evidence that domiciliary care packages can very quickly become more expensive than residential care.

The new system has reduced demand for places in residential care and is accelerating structural changes. Imbalances in the ratio of beds to the local population has led to closures in some areas, while other areas are attracting new entrants. Many smaller homes are finding it difficult to survive with lower occupancy levels and competition from the large companies (Bethel, 1993).

The continued growth of larger public companies has implications for users, authorities and home operators. The provision of large-scale purpose-built homes concentrated in the more heavily populated areas will result in the closure of

Flaws in community care
• Reasons for private care expansion
• Home care can replace care homes

Reality in community care
• No user right of choice
• Home care is not always first choice
• Care homes may be cheaper

Changes in private sector
• Uneven provision is stabilizing
• Closures common
• Growth of corporate providers and their strength
• New demands on home owners/ managers

smaller homes, decreasing choice for users. The corporate operators, with their professional back-up and economies of scale, can also more easily resist costly stipulations by inspectors, thus controlling costs and maintaining competitiveness (Hinchliffe, 1994).

The system of competitive tendering and competition for new clients means that home owners now need negotiation and marketing skills. The tendering process, and the contracting process both impose their own creeping regulations, such as the requirements to have formal policies (on equal opportunities, health and safety and so on), for written procedures to ensure compliance. The small independent operators must become more professional and businesslike, upgrading from a cottage-style industry into a structured business endeavour. Business management skills are needed, together with an awareness of matters such as efficiency, return and investment to retain the confidence of the financial institutions.

Practice point
Private home owners need skills in:
- negotiation
- marketing
- management

THE ROLE OF REGULATION

The registration and inspection process has a major influence on the private sector. While most care providers agree that there is a need for registration and inspection, regulatory problems can operate against the delivery of excellent care. Among these are the sheer quality of often conflicting regulations and guidelines for operation that are issued, the tendency towards overspecification and the lack of assessment of the cost of compliance. The tendency in the guidelines has been towards more and more minute prescription. Registration and inspection officers' insistence that guidelines be followed springs from a misunderstanding of the nature and purpose of guidelines; guidelines are advisory only, they are not mandatory regulations.

Regulation problems
- Excessive
- Conflicting
- Overspecified
- Compliance costs

Staffing ratios provide a prime example of the inflexible manner in which guidelines are imposed and become 'tablets of stone' (Independent Healthcare Association, 1991). The NAHAT supplementary guidelines (1988) state that it is not possible to have standard staffing ratios, (but almost every health authority has such a ratio) and recommends a joint approach to staffing levels between the authority and the nurse in charge. The three good practice steps for joint working – participation, consultation and negotiation – (DoH/KPMG, 1992) – are generally non-existent. Thus staffing levels are normally based on resident numbers rather that on the intensity of activity within the home.

The Department of Health discussion circular on deregulation proposes to examine the registration and inspection processes in the light of these and other factors (Department of Health, 1994). The circular indicated that it is not the function of inspectors to raise standards by imposing unnecessary requirements on owners and managers, and identified that there was a need for guidance on the training of inspectors, particularly as many inspectors have had minimal exposure to this very complex business (Figures 7.1 and 7.2).

It is of even greater concern that the courts have held that inspectors do not have a duty of care to home owners in relation to their actions (*Martine* v. *South East Kent Health Authority*, 1993). There is no procedure for dealing with disputes between inspectors and operators apart from

> **Regulation solutions Department of Health is considering:**
> - reform of registration and inspection
> - clarification of the purpose of inspection
> - training of inspectors

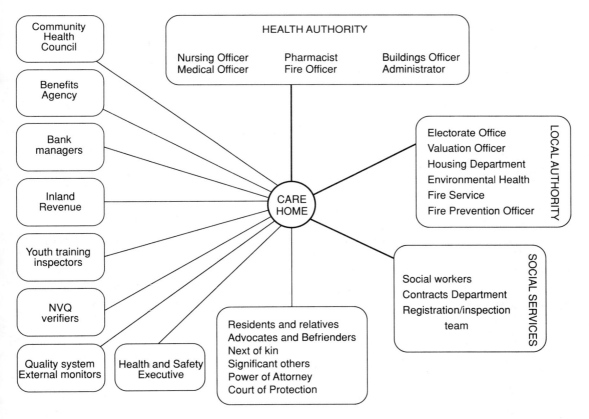

Figure 7.1 Care home stakeholders.

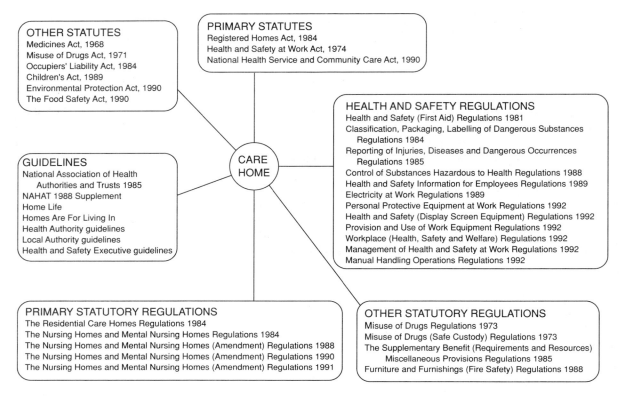

Figure 7.2 Regulation of care homes. Note: this list of statutes and regulations is not, and is not intended to be, exhaustive.

Quality example
The Scottish consultative panel arbitrates between purchasers and providers

proceeding to a costly Registered Homes Tribunal Appeal. However, the publication of reports and the use of lay assessors may help to obtain a more balanced process. The Scottish Home Office and Health Department has established a consultative panel to arbitrate between the health boards and independent hospitals and nursing home operators. Although the panel is not a statutory body and its advice is not legally binding, it is expected that parties will heed its advice and try to resolve their differences accordingly (NHS Management Executive, 1992).

QUALITY ACTIVITIES

The new contracting procedures with local authorities have increased the focus on quality in homes. Although publications such as *Homes are for living in* (DoH/SSI, 1989) seek to address quality of life as an outcome of care, there is still little emphasis on the development of such measures. The registration and inspection processes place very strong emphasis on the more quantifiable aspects of homes, with the implicit assumption that this will lead to higher quality care.

Quality of care is an area that has seen much recent development. Premium payments are available in some areas for homes with quality assurance systems. Indeed, it has been suggested that independently monitored quality schemes could be a basis for reducing inspection procedures (Department of Health, 1994).

The drive for quality, together with the introduction of charters for citizens and patients that emphasize consumer choice, has placed the views of service users centre stage. But quality assurance will not guarantee quality of life nor good care. For example, BS 5750/ISO 9000 is concerned with systemization rather than with the achievement of outcomes such as care plan goals. However, quality activities are an excellent base from which to build good practice into services and management provided they are based on best practice procedures.

Factors promoting quality
• Premium payments
• New quality schemes
• Consumerism

Quality of life – assessing outcome

Obtaining residents' views on the quality of their life (or any other topic) is a very difficult task. Many residents are reluctant to criticize, do not want to complain or cannot envisage an alternative to their current situation (Sinclair, 1988). The traditional questionnaire method of obtaining views is not viable in the care home environment. Detailed interviews are not always possible due to a lack of time or the skills required. Research shows that persevering in obtaining residents' views in a systematic way yields considerable dividends to a home. These include empowerment of residents, participation in active decision making and a sense of taking control over their own lives.

There are several ways of obtaining residents' real views and opinions. Bland offers a useful guide to **interviewing residents** (Bland *et al.*, 1992).

A **residents' forum** to discuss issues such as the daily operation of the home, food, menus and other preferences is a useful step. The forum should be formally established with regular meetings, and minutes taken of the matters discussed and decisions reached. Responsibility for carrying out each action should be identified along with a review date. An

Assessing resident satisfaction
• Interviews
• Residents' forum
• Key workers
• Advocacy schemes

extension of such a forum could involve the relatives and/or friends of residents (Williams, 1994).

The **key worker** system is a further useful method of ensuring that residents' opinions are known. This approach involves intimate knowledge of the earlier life of the residents and their hopes and aspirations. It also involves being a facilitator for promoting resident participation in the home's activities (Worsley, 1992).

A **befriending** scheme, based on advocacy, is another useful option. This may be particularly suitable for residents who have no relatives or regular social contacts. The essence of the scheme is that the friend or advocate speaks on behalf of the resident. If the befriender knew the resident before admission, he/she will be better aware of the resident's views. If not, the advocate would have to befriend the resident to try to ascertain the resident's views. This is a more independent approach than the key worker system (Woolrych, 1990).

Uncovering residents' real views assists in solving the core dilemmas in all residential care homes between the basic values contributing to the quality of life of residents and the operational requirements of running a home (Table 7.1) (Garland, 1991). For example, a resident might wish to sleep undisturbed, yet his/her care plan may call for regular turning. A resident might wish to remain isolated in his/her room, but is that wise if he/she suffers from depression? Consider

Table 7.1 Examples of common dilemmas in establishing basic values

Value	For	Against
Privacy	Right to single room	Isolation in room, withdrawal, depression, cost, monitoring
Dignity	Resident involved in decisions on own care	Antisocial behaviour preventing input
Independence	Facility to make snacks when inclined	Problem of catering and food hygiene regulations
Choice	Use of own furniture	Problem of compliance with fire safety regulations
Rights	Association by choice	Community living sacrifices
Fulfilment	Facilities to use mental and physical faculties	Problem of unwillingness to be active or sociable

that life in residential homes has been the subject of much unfavourable comment (Godlove, Richard and Rodwell, 1982). Much time is spent in lounges watching television or apparently doing nothing. Activities organized by the home are seen as an antidote to this apparent inactivity. However, there is considerable difficulty in straddling the line between persuasion and pressure to join in an activity. And, of course, inspection reports often give insufficient emphasis to activities because the process is not a suitable medium for uncovering residents' wishes, desires and aspirations.

Ultimately, residents' overall satisfaction will depend on the balance between the actual experience of living and prior expectations (Figure 7.3). If the resident has low expectations it may be relatively easy for a home to yield a high level of satisfaction, and vice versa.

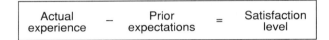

Figure 7.3 Residents' overall satisfaction with a home.

Quality schemes

There is a growing number of schemes and sources of advice in this area. Inside Quality Assurance is a package produced by the Department of Government, Brunel University, that focuses on the ways in which people within a home attempt to understand what quality of life means to them and how they try to achieve that quality. The package evolved from the Department of Health funded Caring in Homes initiative (Youll and McCourt-Perring, 1993).

The Counsel and Care report *Not Only Bingo* surveys a wide range of creative and recreational activities (Birch *et al.*, 1993). The report also suggests good practice measures, such as designating one person to be responsible for the activities programme and how to involve residents and their relatives in planning the programme.

A number of other innovative approaches to activities have been developed during the past few years.

- The writer-in-residence project: a professional writer helped residents with dementia to express their thoughts and memories (Westminster Health Care, 1994).
- Drama therapy can be an effective way of working with people with dementia (Hodgkinson, 1994).

- Photography: this can promote positive images of residents' lives (Crimmens and Kelly, 1994).
- A multimedia project: this was conceived and managed by Artlink and produced an exhibition of photographs together with a video and radio play.
- The Elderly Accommodation Counsel special art award to celebrate the achievement of the over-60s encourages artistic talent (latent or otherwise).
- The Dark Horse Venture aims to discover the hidden talents of older people through recognizing personal achievement.

Quality of care

There has been little research on the relationship between quality of life and quality of care. Since they may be independent of each other, they should not necessarily be taken as proxies for each other. However, quality of care indicators can promote those values that are universally agreed to enhance quality of life. The central issues in quality of care are:

- What is to be measured?
- How is it to be measured?
- Who is to set the standards?

Quality examples
- Department of Health
- The CARE scheme
- Home Life
- Homes are for living in
- Worcester SCAPA

Again, there are a number of approaches and these are available for off-the-shelf purchase. The emphasis in each tends to vary with their origin, and it is often possible to combine various systems to meet the needs of the home.

- The Department of Health has indicated that the presence/absence of pressure sores is an excellent indicator of quality of care (Department of Health, 1993). It suggests that this may help to inform the contracting process between purchasers and providers of services. The report contains a step-by-step approach to tackling the problem, and lists a number of examples of good practice together with contact names and addresses for more information on the case studies.
- The Royal College of Physicians CARE (continuous assessment review and evaluation) scheme is based on key indicators of the quality of care (Table 7.2). The scheme consists of ready-made audits for staff to carry out. Staff enjoy using it and it improves the quality of care (Royal

Table 7.2 Royal College of Physicians Key indicators of quality of care

- Preserving autonomy
- Promoting urinary continence
- Promoting faecal continence
- Optimizing drug use
- Managing fails and accidents
- Preventing pressure sores
- Optimizing the environment, equipment and aids
- The medical role in long-term care

College of Physicians, 1992; Brocklehurst and Dickinson, 1995).

- *Home Life: A Code of Practice for Residential Care* provides a check list of 218 points covering staff, buildings, admission, administration, health care, diet, food and offices (Avebury Working Party, 1984) (revised 1992).
- *Homes are for living in*, although looking at quality of life indicators, includes a series of questionnaires that staff could use for quality audits (DoH/SSI, 1989).
- The Worcester System SCAPA (Standards of Care and Practice Audit) developed by Worcester Health Authority is aimed at self-audit within a nursing home environment and concentrates on general administration issues with sections on the physical, psychological and social needs of residents.
- Investors in People (Moorfoot, Sheffield) is a national scheme for the training and development of staff. It is a benchmark against which employers can measure their progress in this area.
- There is a wide range of proprietary systems ranging from consumer-based systems to those aimed at achievement of ISO 9000.

The cost of implementing proprietary quality systems has been seen as prohibitive for many home operators. Nevertheless, every home can and should establish its own quality system, remembering that any system should provide a flexible framework to build on the existing knowledge of the home's staff and ensure that there is consistency of care around the clock. Often the introduction of quality into the culture of the home is just as important as the means of achieving that quality (Clements and Zarkowska, 1994).

> **Quality scheme**
> Every home should have one

TRAINING

The focus on training encouraged by the community care legislation has seen a growth in the number of homes that have staff members working towards National Vocational Qualifications (NVQs). There is some evidence that purchasers of care recognize NVQs as a positive contribution to quality assurance. For example, Birmingham Social Services Department is paying a premium for nursing homes that have a defined proportion of their care staff registered for NVQs. Working towards NVQs encourages staff to be more responsive to residents' needs. There is also evidence that staff with NVQs need less hands-on supervision, thus releasing senior staff for strategic activities (Joseph Rowntree Foundation, 1994a).

The cost of the NVQ programme is often beyond the resources available to small homes (Joseph Rowntree Foundation, 1994b); nevertheless, even the smallest home can and should set up its own in-house training scheme, perhaps using the framework of Investors in People.

Acquiring skills in the practical care tasks is now very important and is sometimes a health and safety requirement. Skills do not come naturally and must be practised. A simple solution would be to link training topics to the drafting of written procedures. These could then double as training notes and induction aids. In many cases the local Training and Enterprise Council can provide advice, information and resources for training. There is also a number of off-the-shelf training packages of varying quality, scope and cost available. Before selecting a training package, a decision should be made on what is expected from the package, the areas it should cover and the maximum cost.

DIVERSIFICATION OF CARE

The creation of a mixed economy of care was originally anticipated to create a situation in which the private sector would develop new forms of provision and diversity to offer domiciliary services because of several factors.

- The voluntary and private providers would operate with the statutory agencies to achieve greater flexibility.
- There was oversupply of care home places in some areas.
- Client numbers would be further reduced by diversion into home care.

- The effect of the operation of the Special Transitional Grant (STG); 85% of which has to be spent in the private sector.

This diversification ought to have proceeded relatively smoothly given that the STG guaranteed a pool of funding to underpin service provision. In practice, this has not occurred and this is illustrated by discussing four new ways of delivering care.

Domiciliary care

A lack of service providers in the private sector has made it difficult for some authorities to purchase such services. In practice there are three brakes on entry into the domiciliary services market.

- The tension between being a principal service provider or an agent in the supply of personnel to carry out the service. Being an agency reduces the costs and allows competitive bidding.
- The number of hours required to make the service provision viable. Economies of scale are not reached until the service provider is providing between 800 and 1000 hours of care per week.
- The skills of care home owners are very different from the skills required to operate a domiciliary care business.

Outreach services

A second area of diversification is outreach services, which can take a number of forms.

- One authority supplies a personal care service which is delivered locally in residential homes through outreach workers who use the home's facilities to deliver their own care package.
- Some private sector homes are providing meals on wheels on a small scale. The meals are cooked with the meals for the home and are then delivered by a care assistant. This is a local solution to a dispersed rural client base and is not a widespread form of diversification.

Care villages

The care village is an American concept that is aimed at providing care on one site for elderly people through every

---

The slowing of development of Domiciliary care
- Mode of operation
- High cost of low volume
- Different skills required

Outreach seminars
- Low demand

Care villages
- Philosophy clash

Respite care
- High cost
- Purchasing difficulties

stage of old age from full mobility to death. The concept is totally contrary to the thinking behind the community care policy with its emphasis on enabling people to live as independently as possible in the general community (Cm 849, 1989). Concern has been expressed about the dangers of such villages becoming dumping grounds for elderly people – a modern form of institutionalization (Shreeve, 1994).

Respite care

Respite care was another area that promised much in terms of diversification possibilities but has not borne fruit. There are problems of both supply and demand that have not been resolved. Purchasers will not commit to a 52-week contract for respite care because they must demonstrate value for money; a bed place that is contracted for a year and remains empty for part of the year is considered a waste of resources. Purchasers prefer to make spot purchases of respite care, but the resident's right to choose a home and the operation of the assessment system are difficult to fit into the planning process.

On the provider side, respite care without a 52-week contract is not particularly attractive. The throughput of respite residents requires considerably more administration, and the level of care required consumes more resources until the resident becomes known to the staff. Where occupancy levels are good, it is difficult for purchasers to move quickly enough to take up availability, so providers may tend to hedge their bets and wait for a potential long-term resident.

Major challenges
- Service range
- Funding
- Regulation

CURRENT ISSUES

Three major interrelated issues need to be dealt with rapidly – the range of services, funding and regulation.

Range of services

A mixed economy of care will not be achieved quickly. The current (and anticipated) financial difficulties of a number of local authorities (December 1994), together with the ongoing restructuring of the private care sector, will continue to cause disarray in planning. This will prevent market consolidation for some time to come. The cost of refurbishing local authority Part III homes will mean significant numbers of closures, further reinforcing the division between the purchaser and the provider. Demand for places in residential homes will rise due to:

- the growth in the number of dependent elderly people in the population
- the accompanying growth in numbers of disabled and dementia sufferers
- the increase in the number of elderly people living alone
- the reduction in the potential pool of carers.

The problems for home owners of diversification into domiciliary care were outlined above. The cost of supplying home care packages, linked to the pressure on local authority funds and the cost effectiveness of residential care, will quite quickly set a limit to the expansion of this market. There may be a growth in supply of other services but this is more likely to reflect local needs rather than national trends.

The restructuring of the national and local markets will see an increase in smaller specialist units in niche markets. For example, Peugeot Motors is planning a day care centre in Coventry for its workers' elderly relatives. This will further blur the distinction between social and health care. Perhaps the issue will cease to be whether there will be a single type of care home, and will revolve more around the issue of the resources that are required for a needs-led service. In this regard, there has been consistent underappreciation of the input of trained nurses. The symptoms of this undervaluation are the debates about the issues of 'social v. health care' and the skill mixes of public health nursing teams. Often the real input from nurses is difficult to demonstrate since a major part of their skills lie in preventive measures and in carrying out the assessments necessary to maintain health, rather than treat illness. It is often forgotten that the goal of good nursing care is quality of life and not quality of care.

The issue of the corporate providers is also linked to the restructuring of markets. Quite aside from the issues related to choice outlined above, there is a requirement for a political decision to decide at what point there is an equilibrium in the market between the larger and smaller homes sufficient to maintain a balance between choice and cost-effectiveness.

The residential care sector must become a positive choice, as envisioned by the Wagner Report (1988), on the grounds of its innate benefits for residents (24-hour care at a standard higher than could be achieved by living in the community) and its cost-effectiveness.

New forces are
• Long-term care insurance
• Self-financing

Funding

Although the community care legislation changed the system of funding of residential care, it is an incomplete solution to the burgeoning cost of care, because the rapid growth in the elderly population, together with greater levels of dependency, were not taken into account. The private sector will continue to expand, but this growth will now be fuelled by self-financing residents arising from two sources. First, the increasing number of people with long-term care insurance, and second, the rising proportion of people with substantial capital assets (mainly in the form of property).

Regulation and deregulation

Up to now the residential care sector has been viewed with different perspectives (Fig. 7.4). Central government is concerned with regulation and cost. The public sector concentrates on regulation/guidelines and quality, and tends to avoid the issue of cost-effectiveness. The private sector emphasizes the quality of care it supplies cost-effectively, but sees regulation and bureaucracy as a fetter on its operations. The importance of taking an overall rather than a parochial view of residential care should be emphasized.

The current Department of Health discussion paper (Department of Health, 1994) should ensure that the function of registration and inspection is clarified. This, together with training of inspectors should ensure that issues of cost are realistically inserted into the inspection process and that overspecification is curbed. It should also ensure that regulation becomes more acceptable to the private sector by focusing on quality issues.

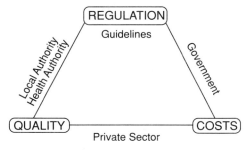

Figure 7.4 Different perspectives on the residential care sector.

CONCLUSION

For many reasons the NHS has failed to deliver high quality long-term care for elderly people. Current trends indicate that the NHS, based as it is on a medical model in which cure is the criterion for success, will continue to withdraw from long-term care. The private sector has expanded and will expand further to fill that gap in provision. It has made a very substantial and often unappreciated contribution to excellent care for elderly people. It has shown itself to be in the forefront of the quality debate and has much to offer in the way of good and innovative practice. It consistently delivers cost-effective, good quality care.

The private sector has earned the right, on its own merits, to be treated as a full and equal partner in the provision of high quality care for elderly people. The substantial shift in perception and evaluation of the private sector that has already begun, must continue.

The issue of funding affects not only the private sector. The major question facing the electorate and politicians is whether they are prepared to support the level of service and resources required to fulfil the needs of our ageing population. An open, honest and informed public debate is essential to establish what level of financing is required to support the appropriate level of service and how that financing should be raised. Underfunding and overspecification can only coexist with service provision at the expense of quality and choice.

REFERENCES

Audit Commission (1988a) *Making a Reality of Community Care*, HMSO, London.

Avebury Working Party (1984 revised 1992) *Home Life: A Code of Practice for Residential Care*, Centre for Policy on Ageing, London.

Bethell, J. (1993) City nurses: an interest in caring for the elderly. *Sunday Times*, 3 October.

Birch, A., Cylwick, H., Elkington, G. *et al.* (1993) *Not Only Bingo*, Counsel and Care, London.

Bland, R., Cheetham, J. *et al.* (1992) *Residential Homes for Elderly People: Their Costs and Quality*, The Scottish Office, HMSO, London.

Brocklehurst, J. and Dickinson, E.J. (1995) The impact of the CARE scheme on the quality of long term care, *Quality in Health Care* (submitted).

Clark, J. (1992) *The Value of Nursing*, Royal College of Nursing, London.

Clements, J. and Zarkowska, E. (1994) *Care Staff Management: A Practitioner's Guide*, John Wiley & Sons, London.

Cm 849 (1989) *Caring for People: Community Care in the Next Decade and Beyond*, HMSO, London.

Crimmens, P. and Kelly, A. (1994) Our greatest resource is ourselves. *Health Service Journal*, **27 October**, 15.

Department of Health/Social Services Inspectorate (1989) *Homes are for Living In*, HMSO, London.

Department of Health/KPMG (1992) *Implementing Community Care – Improving Independent Sector Involvement in Community Care Planning*, DoH, London.

Department of Health (1993) *Pressure Sores – A Key Quality Indicator*, HMSO, London.

Department of Health (1994) *Draft Circular on Registration and Inspection of Private Hospitals and Nursing Homes*, DoH, London.

Firth, J. (1987) *Public Support for Residential Care: Report of a Joint Central and Local Government Working Party*, DHSS, London.

Garland, J. (1991) *Making Residential Care Feel Like Home*, Winslow Press, Bicester.

Godlove, C., Richard, L. and Rodwell, G. (1982) *Time for Action: An Observation Study of Elderly People in Four Different Care Environments*, University of Sheffield.

Griffiths, R. (1988) *Community Care: Agenda for Action*, HMSO, London.

Hinchliffe, D. (1994) *Cutting Corners, Risking Lives*, Labour Party, London.

Hodgkinson, J. (1994) The healing magic of stories. *Journal of Dementia Care*, **Sept/Oct**, 11 & 14–15.

Independent Healthcare Association (1991) *Survey of Residential Care and Nursing Home Costs*.

Joseph Rowntree Foundation (1994a) *NVQs in Residential Homes*, Social Care Briefings, JRF, York.

Joseph Rowntree Foundation (1994b) *Independent Organizations in Community Care*, Social Care Research, No 56, JRF, York.

Laing and Buisson (1993) *Laing's Review of Private Healthcare*, Laing and Buisson, London.

Llewellyn, S. (1993) Residential care for the elderly: Dispelling the myths, *Generations Review*, **3**, 5–8.

Martine v. *South East Kent Health Authority* (1993) Unreported judgement, Court of Appeal, 25 February.

NAHAT (1988) *Registration and Inspection of Nursing Homes*, NAHAT, London.

NHS Management Executive Letter (1992) 40, Scottish Office, Edinburgh.

Royal College of Nursing (1987) *Improving Care of Elderly People in Hospital*, Royal College of Nursing, London.

Royal College of Physicians (1992) *High Quality Long-Term Care for Elderly People: Guidelines and Audit Measures*, Royal College of Physicians, London.

Shreeve, M. (1994) Don't fence me in. Report of comments of the Wolverhampton Social Services Director. *Community Care*, 29 September–5 October.

Sinclair, I. (ed.) (1988) Residential care for elderly people, in *Residential Care: The Research Reviewed* (ed. I. Sinclair), NISW, London.

Wagner, G. (1988) *Residential Care: A Positive Choice: Report of the Independent Review of Residential Care*, HMSO, London.

Westminster Health Care (1994) *The Times of Our Lives*, Westminster Health Care, London.

Williams, B. (1994) Listening to patients. *Health Service Journal*, **20**.

Woolrych, R. (1990) *Developing Day Services*, Association of Professions for Mentally Handicapped People.

Worsley, J. (1992) *Good Care Management*, Age Concern, London.

Youll, P.J. and McCourt-Perring, C. (1993) *Raising Voices: Ensuring Quality in Residential Care*, HMSO/Brunel University, London.

Hospital services 8

Peter P. Mayer

EDITORS' INTRODUCTION

This chapter rounds off the section on sectors of care by looking at hospital services. As in other sectors of care, changes in what is done and how it is done are occurring in hospitals. Dr Mayer manages to combine a historical perspective with an up-to-date analysis of present trends.

The chapter is made up of five main parts. After a brief history of how the specialty of geriatric medicine was born, the main changes that have occurred in hospital services for elderly people are described in the context of the challenge presented to this sector. This is followed by a section that explains the major service elements that go to make up a comprehensive hospital service. This touches upon access, acute services, the discharge phase, specialized services (such as stroke units), day hospitals, outreach clinics, respite care, long-term care and health promotion. In considering each, current changes and tensions are uncovered to assist the reader in understanding how hospital services are being shaped. The role of quality activities is described with particular reference to clinical audit and peer review. Finally, a look forward dwells on how positive responses can be made in shifts to community care and appropriate training for all professionals involved in the care of elderly people.

After reading this chapter, you will have a clear view of the development, principles and components of, and controversies in, hospital services for elderly people. What goes on in hospital often seems complicated and disorganized to the outsider. Here Dr Mayer explains the rationale behind what is experienced. This should help readers from other backgrounds understand the philosophy of specialized care of elderly people and the context within which it is developing. This may be particularly helpful in forming effective working relationships and practical approaches to collaboration and co-operation.

Key topics
- History
- Impact of elderly people
- Service elements
- Quality audit and peer review
- Looking forward

Quality Care for Elderly People. Edited by Peter P. Mayer, Edward J. Dickinson and Martin Sandler. Published in 1997 by Chapman & Hall, London. ISBN 0 412 61830 3

HISTORY

There is a long history of interest in the effects of ageing. Maintaining fitness was recognized as far back as the time of Hippocrates as a means of avoiding them. The term 'geriatrics' was coined by Nascher in 1907. In the UK in the late 1940s, Dr Marjorie Warren, a physician at the West Middlesex Hospital, showed that at least one-third of her 714 'incurable' patients were dischargeable, and another third were potentially dischargeable with appropriate diagnosis and therapy.

In 1947, a small group of physicians set up the Medical Society for the Care of the Elderly, later to become the British Geriatrics Society. At that time many physicians were looking after 200 or more elderly patients in very poor conditions, often in the remnants of 19th-century workhouse accommodation. At the inception of the National Health Service (NHS), medical treatment in one Birmingham hospital was described as 'surprisingly good', but only bed-rest and medication were available. Five doctors looked after 1000 bedridden elderly patients, and two nurses cared for 70 patients (of whom 30 might be incontinent) (Hearn, 1987).

Although at that time the care of elderly people was predominantly seen as the preserve of the consultant physician, the specialty of geriatric medicine developed rapidly. After an initial phase of recognizing that people should be assessed before being admitted to a chronic care facility, there was a period in the late 1940s when consultants in geriatric medicine were appointed, preadmission home visits were instituted, and domiciliary visiting services developed. The first day hospital was established by Dr Lionel Cosins in Oxford in 1952 (Williamson, 1994). The first Chair in Geriatric Medicine was established in Glasgow in 1965. Advances in preventive health care developed alongside large departments of geriatric medicine based in acute and non-acute hospitals.

Subsequently, a number of different models of practice have developed, these are described as 'traditional', 'age-related', and 'integrated' (Table 8.1).

Physicians in geriatric medicine have moved from providing a predominantly rehabilitative and custodial service, to increasing involvement in the acute care of elderly people. The main question now seems to be whether geriatricians should return to the general medical fold with a subspecialty interest in rehabilitation and continuing care of elderly people (Andrews and Brocklehurst, 1987).

Recent changes
- Three main models
- Acute care emphasis
- Reduced NHS long-term care

Table 8.1 Models of geriatric medicine practice*

Traditional	Patients selected by non-geriatrician based on assessed or perceived need
Age-related	Everyone above a defined age (65–85 years), often until beds full
Integrated	Multiconsultant teams with shared juniors and joint responsibility for emergency admissions of all ages

*Derived from Royal College of Physicians, 1994b.

Another important change in geriatric medicine has taken it from being a specialty that accepted appropriate referrals but admitted people often after long periods of waiting, with wards providing a very slow moving and 'apathetic' inpatient service, to being a specialty similar to general medicine, where all-comers are admitted, with the abolition of the waiting list and an emphasis on short lengths of stay and appropriate discharge planning.

During the 1960s and 1970s, local health authorities provided a significant proportion of long-term institutional care but, because of changes in the availability of social security funds, in the 1980s there was a rapid expansion of state-funded private and voluntary residential and long-term nursing care. The NHS, which had been a significant provider of continuing care, was no longer so by the early 1990s.

The UK is unique in the complexity and comprehensiveness of its specialized services for elderly people. In other countries, physicians, who may or may not be recognized as specialists in geriatrics, predominantly look after rehabilitation and continuing care services. Within Europe, only the UK, the Republic of Ireland, The Netherlands and Spain recognize geriatrics as a specialty, although general doctors who look after elderly people in institutions in France require a diploma (Grimley Evans, 1994a). Many European countries provide undergraduate and postgraduate specialist training but Castleden (1994), following a visit to Germany, paints a rather more sombre picture of resources and describes only four geriatric services that can be equated to those in the British system. He describes the best services as better than those available in the UK, but says that the status of geriatrics is very low, as it used to be in the UK.

IMPACT OF ELDERLY PEOPLE ON HOSPITAL SERVICES

Factors affecting impact
- Demographic changes
- Costs of care
- Better care

Better care?
- 'Compression' of morbidity
- Prevention
- Diagnosis
- Treatment

Attempting to predict the needs of elderly people into the next century has instigated considerable discussion. The proportion of very elderly people – those aged over 75 years, especially those aged over 85 years – will increase to the end of this century and well into the next. At the same time, there will be a rapid fall in the proportion of middle-aged carers and the number of school-leavers, which may lead to a serious problem in the recruitment of staff for public services.

In 1989, Kenneth Clarke, the then UK Minister of Health, said that over 40% of the NHS budget and 50% of the personal social services budget was spent on people aged over 65 years. Similar changes are occurring at varying rates throughout the world with a potential major impact on health and social care budgets. Costs are expected to continue to increase as the number of elderly people grows.

The demographic effect may be lessened by an increasing compression of illness and disability towards the end of life, by increasingly sophisticated diagnostic techniques leading to less invasive and more accurate analysis of complex disease states, and by improvement in the prevention and treatment of common disabling disorders of old age such as dementia and stroke. Fundamental approaches through technologies such as molecular biology may attack the very foundation of ageing and challenge our concepts of the difference between ageing and illness. Indeed, national long-term care surveys in the USA (Bruster, 1994) indicate a decrease in the proportion of people with disability with age. However, an opposing pressure, shown in other surveys, are peoples increasing expectations.

The common disorders associated with old age (bone disease, arthropathy, vascular disease, Parkinson's disease, dementing illness, fractured neck of femur) are all susceptible to preventive and therapeutic approaches. The increasing ability to intervene in such disorders is now leading to an increasing proportion of the elderly population requiring specialist hospital services, and increasing academic, and therefore research, interest. Gerontology and geriatric medicine are an essential part of the undergraduate medical curriculum, and increasingly, and appropriately, research funding is targeted towards these major disease complexes.

Purchasing of services to combat these disorders – whether by health authorities or, increasingly in the UK, by fundholding general practitioners (GPs) – requires access to accurate and timely information. Access rates to hospital services vary markedly with age, geography, ethnicity and wealth. Increasingly the services need to recognize these inequities and to target resources at specifically deprived groups. Deprivation may be self-imposed because of attitudes, e.g. ageism, cultural or language differences, or as a direct consequence arising out of the disorders and the isolation of very elderly people, e.g. loss of communication skills due to sensory impairment or neurological disorder (Williams, 1994).

Responsibility of purchasers
- Equity
- Communication with users

SERVICE ELEMENTS

Horrocks (1986) first described the components of comprehensive district health services for elderly people arising out of his experiences as Director of the Health Advisory Service (HAS).

The HAS (MacMahon, 1996) will produce a thematic review of elderly services with a particular emphasis on multidisciplinary assessment and the development of quality indicators for continuing care. There is particular concern about the effects of family health services and health authorities amalgamating, the effect of primary care led commissioning and the identification of key areas in rehabilitation and discharge planning.

Access

There has been an increasing emphasis on elderly people needing equity of access to acute hospital services. Elderly people are less likely to be admitted for some acute, especially surgical, problems, spend longer on waiting lists, and may be perceived as 'too frail' for curative intervention (Dunlop, 1993). This view is increasingly being challenged; for example, thrombolysis following myocardial infarction (Royal College of Physicians, 1991) may be more cost-effective in elderly people than in young people, and it is increasingly recognized that interventions such as hip replacements (The Audit Commission, 1995) cataract surgery, carotid endarterectomy and heart valve replacement (Deiwick, 1995) may not only improve the quality of life but may also be cost-effective in health economic terms. Although QALYs (quality of life years) have been challenged as a measure for elderly people, similar quality of life indicators and other measures are of importance in assessing the allocation of resources (Roberts, 1996).

Acute services

Emphasis on equity has led to proposals for changes in the way specialists in geriatric medicine work within acute hospitals. Traditionally they have run separate services taking patients who have previously been assessed by general physicians and acute specialists.

During the 1970s and 1980s age-related services were developed in the UK in which geriatricians played their full role in the admission of ill elderly people with acute medical conditions, but with an age barrier that varied according to local resources from age 65 to 75 or more. The intention was that these services would provide acute care for all ill elderly people within a particular age group, plus small numbers of people of younger ages who were seen as having needs that required the specialist intervention of a geriatrician. This view has been challenged because services for elderly people were often less well resourced than their sister general medical services, and were often seen as being staffed by people who had not 'made the grade' in acute general medicine. Public perception of such services was that they were still housed in, and were equivalent to 19th-century workhouse services (McLean *et al.*, 1994).

There has therefore been a strong movement for a return to the position at the inception of the NHS in 1948 of integrated general and geriatric medicine. A variety of patterns has been proposed depending on local circumstances and the ability of local physicians to work together. The minimum requirement for such a service is for a single admission system for adults that is based on medical need, not age. People may come in through a specialized admissions unit and then be referred to acute medical or rehabilitation services on or off the district general hospital site. There is a danger that specialist skills in caring for elderly people will atrophy leading to a deterioration in the service to elderly people with non-acute needs, as well as to a loss of teaching skills (Grimley Evans, 1994).

Arguments against separate specialized services
- Worse resources
- Perceived clinical inferiority
- Public association with the workhouse

Practice point
Main principle of integration is a single access point

Measures to show that people are accessing services such as the coronary care unit (The Audit Commission, 1995) and have access to treatments such as thrombolysis and surgical interventions as well as appropriate access to multidisciplinary teams with specialist expertise, need to be developed. Provider units need to agree clear guidelines or protocols with purchasers, and appropriate audits need to be in place to ensure not only equity of access, but that access is appropriate to the needs of the elderly person. There is a danger that 'futile' interventions will fritter away resources an easily as non-interventions. Specialist skills may be needed not only to ensure that interventions are achieved where appropriate, but to prevent futile and inappropriate actions. For example, there has been debate about the role and appropriateness of cardiopulmonary resuscitation within specialist elderly care hospitals. Services such as the Health Advisory Service have pressurized units to carry the full range of resuscitation equipment including defibrillators as well as trained staff. As yet, there is little research to support this potentially costly development (Dickinson, 1991), although ethical arguments may be an important reason for establishing such services. The opportunity cost needs to be clearly evaluated (Davies, King and Silas, 1993).

The admission system should lead to appropriate placement of people within facilities that are likely to achieve the most effective outcomes. There is evidence that 'misplaced' elderly people within the hospital sector have poorer outcomes in terms of both morbidity and mortality. People with the disorders most appropriate to the specialty of geriatric medicine, e.g. stroke, confusion, falls and loss of self-care abilities, will have a longer length of stay in non-specialist services and will often be seen as 'bed-blockers', i.e. someone who stays in a resource longer than deemed appropriate for that resource and for reasons outside the control of those providing the service (Whittaker and Tallis, 1992).

Practice point
Services need to be organized to place patients appropriately

The discharge phase

National guidelines (HC 89(5), DoH, 1989) directed that appropriate discharge arrangements be made for the most vulnerable sectors of the population. This led to an increased emphasis on multidisciplinary planning of discharge (Table 8.1) from the time of admission, the establishment of discharge checklists for monitoring and the role of the local

Discharge developments
• Multidisciplinary planning
• Monitoring checklists
• Liaison with community services

Table 8.2 Good discharge planning

- Provision of appropriate information to patients and carers.
- Appropriate timely communication with other services, including the patient's general practitioner, at least 24 hours before discharge.
- Ensure patient's capacity to manage at home by appropriate predischarge assessments.
- Check fitness of patient on day of discharge.
- Ensure support is available on return (i.e. do not discharge on a Friday!).
- Follow-up information and support available
- Contingency planning
- Reappraisal

Derived from Main (1994).

Moving the setting of care
- Early discharge schemes
- Home support care
- Hospital at home

authority social worker as case manager for the most complex problems (DoH, 1994).

There has been increasing emphasis on the need for discharge to take place only when community support services are agreed and available. Primary care and community-based teams, as well as service users, are encouraged to take part in the process, to monitor the outcome, and to give feedback on the results (Jones and Lester, 1994). 'Exception monitoring' where the system has failed, highlights the worst problems, but the best services provide more comprehensive and regular monitoring including regular monitoring of patient satisfaction to ensure that the process is truly of good quality. Readmission rates are probably the most commonly used indicator, but they are open to perverse incentives, and in the UK are only a record of people readmitted to the unit from which they were discharged (Williams and Fritter, 1988) (Table 8.2).

Various hospital services have developed schemes that support ill or dependent people on discharge, both as a means of shortening the length of hospital stay as well as decreasing the impact of severe illness and disability on people's return to their own homes. Various projects have shown that the input of high intensity support for the most vulnerable and disabled elderly people immediately following discharge from hospital may, in the long-term, decrease the need both for readmission and support services (Martin, Oyewole and Moloney, 1994). Hospital at home schemes were pioneered for patients who had experienced traumatic injury. They have since been developed and become available for other patients. These schemes have shown the possibility of providing high quality intensive specialized support at home for a small number of people with appropriate home circumstances (Costain and Warner).

Specialized services

Geriatric orthopaedic services have become an established part of UK health practice (Reid, 1994). There is evidence to support improved outcomes for vulnerable elderly people who are jointly managed, but there are some concerns about the cost effectiveness of such services if the rehabilitation unit is on a different site from the surgical unit. Elderly people who have suffered major trauma, especially fractured neck of femur, are often very frail and outcomes very poor, and there may be difficulty in judging whether these units are best used for people with a potentially good outcome or for those with the most complex problems (Farnworth, Kenny and Shiell, 1994). Standardized Assessment Scales may assist in identifying good outcomes (Shepherd, 1996).

Stroke units and dedicated teams within acute and non-acute settings improve patient outcomes. Acute units' main focus is on early intervention with accurate diagnosis plus, increasingly, on medication. Non-acute stroke units' major function is rehabilitation where similar questions to those concerned with orthopaedic rehabilitation must be answered. Meta-analysis has confirmed the effectiveness of such interventions (Langhorne *et al.*, 1993).

The skills needed for multidisciplinary rehabilitation are increasingly recognized as a specialist skill in geriatric medicine, and there is increasing evidence of effectiveness for both in and out patients (Young, 1995).

These services increasingly recognize the need for the hospital to be outward looking, and they view successfully establishing back into the community people who have disorders whose ramifications last well beyond the bounds of the acute illness, as part of their responsibility. Mortality rates in elderly care units are usually fairly low but many have developed palliative care services. Whether such services should be provided in a hospital as an outreach service or as a purely community-based service with appropriate support to allow people to die in their own homes, needs further exploration (Thorpe, 1993).

Practice point
• Orthogeriatric services
• Stroke units
• Palliative care
• Psychiatry of old age

Key trends
- Community emphasis
- Behavioural therapy
- Strong intersector links

Until recently, psychiatric services for elderly people in the UK were part of the general psychiatric services and focused heavily on those requiring long-term institutional care within large peripheral hospitals. With the establishment of a specialist service, there has been an increasing emphasis on providing support to people in their own homes rather than in institutions. Psychiatric services in the UK are increasingly being moved out of the hospital sector, except for assessment and diagnosis, and being provided through day centres, community-based mental health clinics and the development of specialist roles such as the community psychiatric nurse. The psychiatric service of the future is likely to have only a small hospital base, although a large number of elderly mentally disabled people will be admitted to the general medical and geriatric medical sectors of the hospital service, either for intercurrent illness or because of problems in the community.

Access to specialist intervention at home is essential to prevent inappropriate admissions. Again, there needs to be clear monitoring of 'misplacement', and not only the effects of missed diagnoses (Bowler, 1994) on the service user, but the effects of their behaviour on other service users, especially in the acute hospital setting. Inappropriate administration of tranquillizers in response to disturbed behaviour on an acute ward constitutes an assault on the individual, and their misplacement is a potential problem for others. One of the commonest complains from patients in geriatric medical units is about the disturbed behaviour of other patients.

The Excellent Care Awards in the West Midlands (WMIGM, 1993) found many examples of excellent specialized care of elderly people in mental illness services; the aims of these services varied from assessment to relief, but all were based on an effective multidisciplinary team with strong links across the hospital/community boundary and a recognition that even the most disorientated person has areas of ability. Techniques such as reality orientation and reminiscence therapy are used to assist orientation. The most extreme example of this is an elderly care unit in the Bolingbroke Hospital where the environment can be changed to fit in with the type of environment a person lived in when younger (*Sunday Times*, 1989). St Matthew's Hospital at Burntwood used a day care unit for inpatients to maintain abilities by contact with community patients who also attended. These units express the best team practice. As the St Chad's Unit in Stafford puts it: 'We try to see people in a "whole" setting and to do this we must run as a "whole": all pulling together for the same cause to serve our patients as fully as we can.'

Day hospitals

Day hospitals have become an important part of geriatric medical and psychiatric practice. Their functions vary but they mainly provide a base for active or maintenance rehabilitation of physically disabled elderly people within the geriatric medical sector or mentally disabled people within the psychiatric sector. There has been increasing concern about the role of the former, which were established to accelerate the discharge process and to help maintain people in their own homes. People often spend a considerable amount of time travelling (transport therapy) and spend a relatively short period actually at the day hospital for therapy.

Purchasers are increasingly concerned with looking at alternative, relatively less costly, methods of intervention (Young and Forster, 1993). The Royal College of Physicians has published standards and audit measures on the management of day hospitals (RCP, 1994a, 1994b). Unfortunately these resources have become caught up in a futile discussion about health and social needs because, in the UK, the former services are free, and the latter are charged for. In these circumstances, which may affect the community more than the hospital services, the inequity of differential funding, and service delivery arrangements based on a concept that bears little relation to the needs of elderly people, can lead to a severe deterioration in the delivery of an appropriate quality of care.

Joint purchasing arrangements for the development of a consortium of providers may be one way of tackling this problem. At a minimum, day hospitals need to be accessible to everyone likely to benefit from multidisciplinary rehabilitation: this requires flexible transport services to facilitate attendance for the treatment required, and prevention of people having to spend long periods without active intervention.

These services, like beds within hospital, should be used for the appropriate length of time to achieve agreed outcomes, and discharge planning is as important in this sector as in inpatient services. The best day hospitals provide access to all adult age groups, have minimal barriers to referral and provide a wide range of services, some within and some reaching out from the facility.

> **Practice point**
> Day hospitals are a microcosm of wider controversies:
> * philosophically sound – a hospital/community bridge
> * hard to organize
> * uncertain cost-effectiveness
> * opportunity for imaginative development
> * ideal community link

Day hospitals are the shop windows of the specialized hospital services and are sites for demonstrating the particular skills provided by elderly care services. Dedicated services such as falls clinics, memory clinics, continence services, skin care services including specialized approaches to leg ulcers, ideally link with services provided by primary care and local authority sites. The day hospital at the George Eliot Hospital in Nuneaton has given the best service over 10 years of the Excellent Care Awards, demonstrating many features including good co-ordination of care, and continuous evaluation and assessment based on individual need with the aims of maximizing physical independence, and mental and emotional stability. It is twinned with a French hospital, which staff visit, and the service itself provides access to a wide variety of disciplines. The inpatient service is fully integrated.

Below is a poem written by a grateful patient.

An ode to the ladies in charge, Cheverel Wing Day Hospital, George Eliot Hospital

To Sister, Ann, Wendy, and all the other nurses, whose
names I do not know
Just before Christmas I suffered a stroke,
A frightening thing, believe me no joke,
they rushed me to hospital because I could not move,
there they worked on my body to try to improve,
then when I got some movement back,
they sent me home, I had got the sack.
As I sat there in grief and pain,
a letter from the hospital came,
from the people there to say,
come to the hospital each Tuesday.
Off I went in wonderment,
wondering what this letter meant,
a lovely nurse met me at the door,
to make me feel at home, I'm sure,
asked my name, took me to a seat,
brought me a lovely cup of tea,
did all sorts of tests,
then took me to join the rest.
There they asked would I like a game,
to pass the time 'til the dinner came, then the physios came
our limbs to stretch,

to make us feel much better yet,
so Sister, nurses and all helpers too,
thank you all and God bless you.

From one most grateful person, speaking for others, the ladies, Les, Reg, Bill and me, etc.

Outreach clinics

There has also been some development of outreach specialist services in health centres and community hospitals (Bailey, Black and Wilkins, 1994). Consultant clinics for specialties such as obstetrics, dermatology and hearing impairment have been well described. There has been less experience of such services provided by specialist elderly care medicine and are better described in old age psychiatry. Whether the increased access of primary care staff and patients is balanced by the loss of the specialist to the hospital service has not been demonstrated and needs further exploration. It has been suggested that effective follow-up can be undertaken by telephone for some people (Rao, 1994).

Respite care

Respite care services have developed across the whole spectrum of agencies and include services such as Crossroads Care, which provides care in patients' own homes, to hospital-based services, which vary from the provision of care for a few days in each week for the most disabled people, to periods of a week or two once a year to cover carers' holidays (Harman and Naylor, 1985). The best services are flexible, responding to need when requests are made or booked to suit the requirements of patients and their carers (Nolan and Grant, 1992). The Community Care Act, 1990 has focused purchasers' attentions on the criteria for people requiring such services within the NHS, and whether such services should be provided *ad hoc* or within dedicated units (Mayer, 1988). A recent winner of the Excellent Care Award is Moseley Hall Hospital, Birmingham, which provides a service that includes inpatient beds in a special unit, day care, satellite units within residential homes and multidisciplinary teams that can visit people at home to assess them and to provide support services. Arguably its greatest success has been its ability to work alongside community-based services and move that much nearer to achieving 'seamless' care.

Long-term care

During the 1980s, people requiring long-term institutional care were increasingly managed outside the NHS. Central guidance has re-established the role of the NHS in funding or providing long-term institutional care (NHS Executive, 1994). Standards for the management of people within statutory and non-statutory care have been published through the Royal College of Physicians and an audit programme has been described (RCP/BGS, 1992 and studied). Standards need to be established across the statutory, private and voluntary sectors (Harwood and Ebrahim, 1994). For patients in hospital the care management procedure is part of the discharge planning process, and access to statutory or non-statutory services needs to be appropriate and based on need rather than financial or other non-clinical or non-social criteria.

Despite ministerial emphasis on choice and positive outcomes of research into NHS nursing homes, individuals often have little choice. There is a lack of appropriate non-statutory providers and access to free NHS facilities is strictly limited (Henwood, 1992). The corollary of these developments is that the dependency levels within the statutory long-term care sector is very high (Wood and Castledon, 1993).

Publication of a White Paper on Continuing Health Care Needs (DoH, 1995) places firm responsibilities on the NHS to fund long-term health care and a Health Committee Report (1996) looks at options such as only funding the nursing element, and at insurance schemes to offset the costs.

Health promotion

Health promotion
- much needed
- underdeveloped
- being supported by the health promoting hospital initiative

There is a marked variation in life expectancy in the developed world, and the UK has a relatively poor record. There is a need for development of preventive health measures as expressed in the Ottawa Charter (1986). The British Geriatrics Society (1993) policy indicates the areas where preventive techniques may be applicable to very elderly people, with the potential for major impacts as vascular disorders, cancer, mental illness and accidents. Access to relevant services may be through the primary health care team, e.g.

the community geriatrician may lead to competition between the primary and secondary care sectors as service providers to elderly people (Roland, 1996).

REFERENCES

Age and Ageing (1994) The role of the physician in geriatric medicine in the ageing society. *Age and Ageing* (supplement), **3**.

Andrews, K. and Brocklehurst, J. (1987) *British Geriatric Medicine in the 1980s*, King Edward's Hospital Fund, London.

The Audit Commission (1991) *Acute Hospital Care*, Audit Commission, London.

The Audit Commission (1991) *The Virtue of Patients: making best use of nursing resources*, Audit Commission, London.

The Audit Commission (1995) *Dear to Our Hearts? Commissioning Services for the Treatment and Prevention of Coronary Artery Disease*, HMSO.

The Audit Commission (1995) *United They Stand. Co-ordinating Care for Elderly Patients with Hip Fracture*, HMSO.

Bailey, J., Black, M.E. and Wilkins, D. (1994) Specialist outreach clinics in general practice. *British Medical Journal*, **308**, 1053–6.

Bowler, C. (1994) Detection of psychiatric disorders in elderly medical in-patients. *Age and Ageing*, **23**, 307–11.

British Geriatrics Society (1993) *Health care of elderly people in hospital. Recommendations to purchasers and providers*, BGS, London.

British Geriatrics Society (1993) *Health Promotion in Later Life*, BGS, London.

Bruster, S. (1994) National Survey of Hospital Patients. *British Medical Journal*, **309**, 154–9.

Cape, R.D.T. and Gibson, S.J. (1994) The influence of clinical problems, age and social support on outcomes for elderly persons referred to regional aged care assessment teams. *Australia and New Zealand Journal of Medicine*, **24**, 378–85.

Castleden, C.M. (1994) A visit to Germany. *Journal of the Royal College of Physicians*, **28**, 434–8.

Cole, M.G. (1993) Assessing the effectiveness of geriatric services: a proposed methodology. Canadian Task Force on the Periodic Health Examination. *Candadian Medical Association Journal*, **148**, 939–44.

Costain, D. and Warner, M. (no date) *From Hospital to Home Care*, King's Fund, London.

Davies, K.N., King, D. and Silas, J.H. (1993) Professional attitudes to cardiopulmonary resuscitation in departments of geriatric and general medicine. *Journal of the Royal College of Physicians*, **7**, 127–30.

Deiwick, M., Mollhoff, T., Budde, J. and Scheld, H.H. (1995) Cardiac Surgery in Patients Aged 80 Years and Above: Does Outcome Justify Significant Preoperative Morbidity. *Cardiology in the Elderly*, **3**, 381–6.

Department of Health (1989) *Working for Patients*, CM 555, HMSO, London.

Department of Health (1989) HC 89(5), HMSO, London.

Department of Health (1990) *The Quality of Medical Care*, HMSO, London.

Department of Health (1991) *The Patient's Charter*, HMSO, London.

Department of Health (1994) *Hospital Discharge Workbook. A Manual on Hospital Discharge Practice*, Department of Health, London.

Department of Health (1994) *NHS Day Hospitals for Elderly People in England*, HMSO, London.

Dickinson, E.J. (1991) Resuscitation of elderly patients in current medical literature. *Geriatrics*, **4**, 35–9.

Dunlop, W.E. (1993) Effects of age and severity of illness on outcome and length of stay in geriatric and surgical patients. *Medical Journal of Surgery*, **65**, 577–80.

Dunstan E.J., Amar K., Watt A. and Seymour D.G. (1996) First Steps in Building ACME – An Admission Case Mix System for the Elderly. *Age and Ageing*, **25**, 102–8.

Farnworth, M.G., Kenny, P. and Shiell, A. (1994) Cost and effects of early discharge in the management of fractured hip. *Age and Ageing*, **23**, 190–4.

Green, S. (1992) Outcome measures for the elderly. *International Journal of Health Care Quality Assurance*, **5**, 17–22.

Grimley Evans, J. (1994) High hopes . . . for geriatrics. *Journal of the Royal College of Physicians*, **28**, 392–3.

Harman, D. and Naylor, S.E. (1985) *Give Us a Break*, West Midlands Regional Health Authority, Birmingham.

Harwood, R.H. and Ebrahim, S. (1994) Assessing the effectiveness of audit in long stay hospital care for elderly people. *Age and Ageing*, **23**, 287–92.

Hearn, G.W. (1987) *Dudley Road Hospital 1887–1987*, Dudley Road Hospital, Birmingham.

Henwood, M. (1992) Through a glass darkly. *King's Fund Institute Research Report*, **14**, 29–41.

HMSO (1996) *Long Term Care: Future Provision and Funding*. Health Committee Third Report. Volume 1, HMSO, London.

Homer, A.C. and Gilleard, C.J. (1994) The effect of in-patient care on elderly patients and their carers. *Age and Ageing*, **23**, 274–6.

Hopkins, A. and Costain, D. (1990) *Measuring the Outcomes of Medical Care*, RCP/King's Fund, London.

Horrocks, P. (1986) Components of a comprehensive district health service for elderly people – a personal view. *Age and Ageing*, **15**, 321–42.

Inouye, S.K., Acumporee, D., Miller, R.L. *et al.* (1993) A controlled trial of a nursing-centred intervention for hospitalized elderly medical patients: the Yale Geriatric Care Program. *Journal of the American Geriatrics Society*, **41**, 1353–60.

JAGS (1994) Futility in clinical practice. *Journal of the American Geriatrics Society*, **42**, 861–904.

Jones, D. and Lester, C. (1994) Hospital care and discharge: patients' and carers' opinions. *Age and Ageing*, **23**, 91–6.

King's Fund (1989) *Hospital at Home*, King's Fund, London.

King's Fund (1993) *Medical Audit – Taking Stock*, King's Fund, London.

Langhorne, P., Williams, B.O., Gilchrist, W. and Howie, K. (1993) Do stroke units save lives? *Lancet*, **342**, 395–8.

Ledesert, B., Lombrail, P., Yeni, P. *et al.* (1994) The impact of a comprehensive multi-dimensional geriatric assessment programme on duration of stay in a French acute medical ward. *Age and Ageing*, **23**, 223–37.

MacMahon D.G. (1996) Reviewing Health Services for Elderly People in Making a Mark. The Annual Report of the Director. 1994–95. HAS HMSO.

Main, A. (1994) Quality standards in discharge planning. *Journal of the West Midlands Institute of Geriatric Medicine*, **20**, 32–5.

Marks, L. (1990) *Hospital Care at Home: Prospects and Pitfalls*, King's Fund Institute, London, pp. 106–11.

Marks, L. (1991) *Discharging patients and responsibilities? Acute hospital discharge and elderly people*, King's Fund Institute, London, pp. 113–19.

Martin, F., Oyewole, A. and Moloney, A. (1994) A randomised controlled trial of a high support hospital discharge team for elderly people. *Age and Ageing*, **23**, 228–34.

Mayer, P. (1988) Market research improving services for the elderly, in *Consumer and Market Research in Health Care* (eds M. Luck *et al.*), Chapman and Hall, London, pp. 162–4.

McLean, K.A., Austin, C.H., Neul, K.R. and Charmer, K.S. (1994) Integration between general and geriatric medicine: a needs related policy. *Journal of the Royal College of Physicians*, **28**, 415–8.

NHS Responsibilities for Meeting Continuing Health Care Needs. HSG (95) 8. DoH 1995.

NHSE (1993) *Health Promoting Hospitals*, National Health Service Executive, Leeds.

NHSE (1994) *Improving the Effectiveness of the NHS*, EL(94)74, National Health Service Executive, Leeds.

NHSE (1994) *NHS Responsibilities for Meeting Long Term Health Care Needs*, National Health Service Exuecutive, Leeds.

Nolan, M. and Grant, G. (1992) *Regular Respite*, Age Concern England, London.

Ottawa Charter (1986) The Ottawa Charter for Health Promotion: An International Conference on Health Promotion.

Rao, J.N. (1994) Follow-up by telephone. *British Medical Journal*, **309**, 1527–8.

RCP (1991) *Cardiological Interventions in Elderly Patients*, Royal College of Physicians, London.

RCP (1992) *High Quality Long Term Care for Elderly People: Guidelines and Audit Measures*, Royal College of Physicians, London.

RCP (1994a) *Clinical Audit Scheme for Geriatric Day Hospitals*, Royal College of Physicians, London.

RCP (1994b) *Geriatric Day Hospitals: Their Role and Guidelines for Good Practice*, Royal College of Physicians, London.

Reid, J. (1994) In collaboration with orthopaedic surgeons. *Age and Ageing*, **23**, 531–3.

Roberts, H. and Philp, I. (1996) Prioritising Performance Measures for Geriatric Medical Services: What do the Purchasers and Providers Think. *Age and Ageing*, 326–8.

Roland, M. (1996) Defining Core General Practitioner Services. *British Medical Journal*, **313**, 704.

Shepherd, S.M. and Prescott, R.J. (1996) Use of Standardised Assessment Scales in Elderly Hip Fracture Patients. *Journal of the Royal College of Physicians*, **3**, 335–43.

Stone, S.P. and Whincup, P. (1994) Standards for the hospital management of stroke. *Journal of the Royal College of Physicians*, **28**, 52–8.

Sunday Times (1989) Winning entries for the Best of Health Hospital of the Year awards.

Thorpe, G. (1993) Enabling dying people to remain at home. *British Medical Journal*, **1307**, 915–8.

Trerney, A.J. and Worth, A. (1995) Readmissions of elderly patients to hospital. *Age and Ageing*, **24**, 163–6.

Whittaker, J. and Tallis, R. (1992) Misplaced elderly patients in hospital: clarifying responsibilities. *Health Trends*, **24**, 15–17.

WHO (1991) *Budapest Declaration on Health Promoting Hospitals*, World Health Organization, Geneva.

Williams, E.I. and Fitten, F. (1988) Factors affecting early unplanned readmission of elderly patients to hospital. *British Medical Journal*, **297**, 748–87.

Williams, R. (1994) *Commissioning Services for Vulnerable People*, NHS Health Advisory Services, London.

Williamson, J. (1994) In the past. *Age and Ageing*, **23**, 59–61.

WMIGM (1993) *Excellent Care for Older People 1982–1993. A West Midlands Perspective*, West Midlands Institute of Geriatric Medicine, Birmingham.

Wood, P. and Castledon, M. (1993) Dependency, quality and staffing of institutions for elderly people. *Health Trends*, **25**, 97–101.

Young, J. and Forster, A. (1993) A day hospital and home physiotherapy for stroke patients: a comparative cost-effectiveness study. *Journal of the Royal College of Physicians*, 27, 252–8.

Young, J.B. (1995) Effectiveness of Rehabilitation for Older People. *Current Medical Literature Geriatrics*, 8, 63–7.

Part Three
People

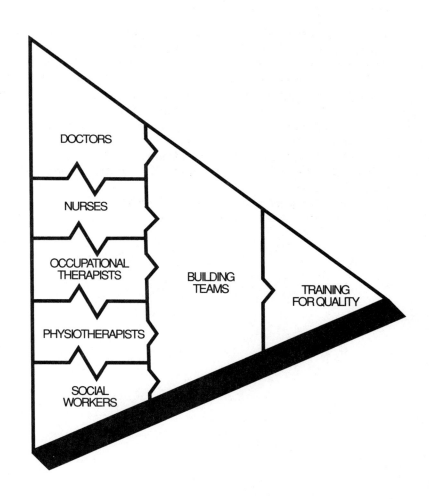

DOCTORS

NURSES

OCCUPATIONAL
THERAPISTS

PHYSIOTHERAPISTS

SOCIAL
WORKERS

BUILDING
TEAMS

TRAINING
FOR QUALITY

EDITORS' INTRODUCTION TO PART THREE

The main pathway to high quality of care is through people, specifically those who deliver care. Unless they are clear on their roles, are valued, trained and moulded into effective teams, high quality is unlikely. As we have seen in the previous part, the sectors of care are different but need to work together in partnership. The same applies to the different disciplines of care.

The purpose of this part is twofold:

- to briefly examine the perspectives of various care disciplines
- to use this as a foundation for considering the specific question of how to develop teams for care and the general role of training.

We expect this part to give the reader insights into the roles of the different disciplines and advice on how to translate these into an effective care team.

Chapter 9 opens this part of the book by examining some of the different disciplines involved in team-based care. The editors acknowledge that many others such as speech and language therapists, hearing therapists, clinical psychologists, dieticians, and continence advisers will also be involved in care from time to time.

Chapter 10 develops the theme of people from different disciplines working together by looking at how to build successful teams.

Chapter 11 widens the discussions of team building to the issue of developing people for their work. This chapter examines training in different disciplines and analyses how this contributes to the quality of care.

By the end of this part, the reader will be aware of the key issues and activities in the main care disciplines and how to develop teams.

The multidisciplinary 9
team

Doctors 9a

Peter P. Mayer and
Edward J. Dickinson

EDITORS' INTRODUCTION

This chapter discusses the role of doctors in promoting high quality care for elderly people. Although the prime responsibility of doctors has traditionally been the diagnosis and treatment of medical conditions, there are several other key roles that doctors undertake. The most important widening of this role lies in its extension beyond the acute organ-based situation to the deployment of knowledge of patterns of chronic disease and disability in the provision of holistic care for elderly people. This is best seen in the specialty of geriatric medicine which is characterized by holistic care, comprehensive care services, interdisciplinary teamwork, managerial interest, relationship building and constant evolution; but many doctors other than specialists are involved in the care of elderly people.

Key topics
- Features of geriatric medicine
- Role of GPs and other specialists
- Role of old age specialists
- Comprehensive services and working in organizations

ROLE OF GPs AND OTHER SPECIALISTS

Doctors look after elderly people in many settings, and may be GPs, specialists in the care of elderly people or specialists in other areas.

- General practitioners: GPs have intimate knowledge of the elderly person, the family and the social situation. They treat the majority of day to day problems as well as performing health promotion and screening activities such as the over 75s checks. More and more GPs have received training in the specialized care of elderly people, and some formalize this by obtaining the Diploma in Geriatric Medicine. The GP has a vital role in the interface with specialist

Features of geriatric medicine
- Holistic
- Comprehensive
- Interdisciplinary
- Managerial
- Relationships

Quality Care for Elderly People. Edited by Peter P. Mayer, Edward J. Dickinson and Martin Sandler. Published in 1997 by Chapman & Hall, London. ISBN 0 412 61830 3

secondary care services, in the wider primary health care team and in liaison with community care services. Many are also trained in other medical specialties such as cardiology or gastroenterology.

- Hospital specialists: many secondary care specialists have a major responsibility for the care of elderly people, e.g. general physicians, orthopaedic surgeons and general surgeons. Despite this, these specialists are unlikely to have been trained in the care of elderly people. Moreover, they are less likely to deliver care in the context of an interdisciplinary team.

ROLE OF OLD AGE SPECIALISTS

Specialists in the care of elderly people include both geriatricians and old age psychiatrists. They are usually hospital-based, although community posts are now emerging. They deal with about 40% of people over the age of 65 years, focusing (through a variety of service models) on those who need their services. These are typically patients who are frail with disability and multiple pathology. They often present with the 'giants' of geriatric medicine – instability, incontinence, immobility, inability, and intellectual impairment. Thus, these specialist physicians have a detailed knowledge of the non-specific presentation of disease, the natural history of old age disorders and the relationships between complex impairments and disability.

COMPREHENSIVE SERVICES

Specialists in the health care of elderly people have been greatly involved in the development of 'comprehensive' services. This has meant the build up of several linked elements such as acute care, rehabilitation, long-term care, outpatient clinics, day hospitals, domiciliary visiting and liaison services for other specialties. The greatest recent changes are the major move of long-term care from NHS to private providers and the increasing involvement in the acute care of elderly people in general hospitals.

The paramount need for teamwork in the care of elderly people is derived from their complex needs. To deliver holistic care, tasks must be delegated among the members of the care team. Here the specialist will certainly contribute diagnostic and therapeutic skills and will often carry out the role of team leader. S/he is trained to be aware of the roles of other team members and may be trained in interpersonal and leadership skills as well. However, teamwork in other specialties and in primary care is less well developed.

WORKING IN ORGANISATIONS

The work of doctors has also been extended to a wider managerial role. Many specialists are now clinical directors, taking the overall responsibility for running a particular specialty. In doing this they are accountable, through the Medical Director, to the Trust Board. Managerial training of specialists is now routine. Indeed many doctors now obtain a formal management qualification such as the Masters in Business Administration. Associated with this managerial interest is the growth of clinical audit, now a required activity for all doctors. What began as **medical** audit, is now moving to become **clinical** audit to reflect the interdisciplinary nature of routine care. Audit may identify a need to change practice, the system of care or the resources used. Many doctors and managers may find such change hard to achieve.

To achieve high quality care, doctors have a key role in building effective external relationships. Since services for elderly people exist in so many settings, doctors have an overarching role as patient advocates in the planning of services, in liaison, and in joint activities. This is an extension of the central doctor–patient relationship, which lies at the core of the practice of medicine. This is now most clearly expressed in the involvement of provider doctors in the commissioning of services. This occurs in two ways. First, commissioners are expected to work with clinicians in developing their commissioning strategies and specifications. Second, GP fundholding has been introduced. In this role doctors need to manage the conflict between providing services for individuals and using resources widely to meet the needs of populations. Physicians who specialize in the care of elderly people seem particularly skilled in handling this dilemma.

Overall, all doctors concerned with the care of elderly people face the exciting challenges of working with colleagues in other specialties, with the other disciplines of the clinical care team, with managerial colleagues and with agencies working in other sectors. Even when the NHS has been free of major

> **Working in organizations**
> - Team care
> - Managerial role
> - Clinical audit
> - Commissioning

reorganization, there has been restless change in the pattern of geriatric medicine services to try and achieve even greater equity, effectiveness and humanity in care.

FURTHER READING

Andrews, K. (1987) *Rehabilitation of the older Adult*, Edwin Arnold, London.

Horrocks, P. (1982) The case for geriatric medicine: an age-related specialty, in *Recent Advances in Geriatric Medicine*, Vol. 2 (ed. B. Isaacs), Churchill Livingstone, London.

Royal College of Physicians of London (1977) *Report of Working Party on Medical Care of the Elderly*, RCP, London.

Royal College of Physicians (1995) *Ensuring Equity and Quality of Care for Elderly People*, RCP, London.

Williamson, J. (1979) Notes on the historical development of geriatric medicine as a medical specialty. *Age and Ageing*, 8, 144–8.

Nurses 9b

Karen A. Luker and
Karen R. Waters

EDITORS' INTRODUCTION

Whatever the setting, the nursing input is omnipresent. The
type of nursing varies depending on the setting, yet the nurse
is often the co-ordinator of the multiprofessional team. This
chapter explores the nursing role and its interaction with the
multidisciplinary teams.

Key topics
- The nurse's role
- A study of teams

THE NURSE'S ROLE

Teamwork in elderly care has been the preferred mode of
practice, especially on rehabilitation wards. Multidisciplinary
teams are complex since the tasks they undertake are varied
and the skills are of differing types and levels (Webb and
Hobdell, 1980).

The way in which this heterogeneous group of people actually discharges its responsibility is intricate and complex.
Although all members may share a broad common goal of
service provision, it is suggested that their individual occupational orientations may lead to differing perspectives and
priorities. The leadership of the team may also affect its
functioning. It is common practice for the consultant physician to take on the role of leader, and while other team
members are recognized as potential leaders of the team,
whether they take on this leadership role depends on the
consultant (Evers, 1981). Concern has been expressed about
whether sufficient attention is paid in practice to the resolution of conflicts and overlapping roles within the team (Evers,
1981; Fairhurst, 1981; Engstrom, 1986).

The nursing role in the multidisciplinary team has been the

Quality Care for Elderly People. Edited by Peter P. Mayer, Edward J.
Dickinson and Martin Sandler. Published in 1997 by Chapman & Hall,
London. ISBN 0 412 61830 3

Table 9b.1   Conceptualization of the nursing role

Core functions	Activities
Ward management	Management and organization of nursing care and nursing team. Management of human and physical resources. Co-ordination of personnel visiting and/or working on the ward. Liaison between team members. Point of contact for relatives/visitors.
Custodial role	Twenty-four-hour presence on ward. Maintenance of patient safety. General responsibility for patients.
Delegated role	Administration of medicines and other treatments.
Specialized role	
General maintenance	Maintenance of patient continence, tissue viability, personal hygiene, ability to dress and move.
Specialist	Prevention and treatment of pressure sores, continence promotion and management.
Carry-on role	Carry on work of therapists, particularly in dressing and walking. Liaison between nurses and therapists.

focus of some attention (e.g. Waters and Luber, 1996), but not fully explored. The nursing role in a ward-based multidisciplinary team might be conceptualized as having core functions that remain the same regardless of the care groups, and a more specialist role that will be shaped by the nature of the patient group. Table 9b.1 highlights the functions in the context of an elderly rehabilitation ward.

The nurse's role is generally viewed as one of co-ordinator of the multidisciplinary team, and manager of the nursing team. This co-ordinating function stems from the 24-hour responsibility for the ward. From the perspective of elderly patients and their carers or significant others, the ward sister or charge nurse is the first point of contact for information and support. A general role relating to the maintenance of daily living activities and general well-being and comfort of the patient has been seen as the business of nurses.

Specialized functions have been ascribed to nurses in elderly care settings, such as tissue viability and continence promotion. In a multidisciplinary setting, where clients are having treatment and in contact with a number of different disciplines, the nurse may assume a 'carry-on' role. For example, nurses carry on the work of therapists in their absence, e.g. walking and dressing practice. This role is very important in the facilitation of independence in elderly people, as therapists are not present in ward settings for over 50% of the patient's waking time.

The Royal College of Nursing document *The Role of the Nurse in the Rehabilitation of Elderly People* defines the following elements of the nursing role within the multidisciplinary team.

- Liaison with relatives and carers
- Initiating contact with other team members
- Giving and receiving information
- Administering prescribed therapy
- Monitoring effects of other therapies
- Reporting back
- Taking part in evaluation
- Assessing clients.

The nursing role can be seen to be multifaceted and potentially different in various settings. There is little empirical evidence available to inform us on the way multidisciplinary teams function in elderly care. Some research has been undertaken in the primary health care field, but with respect to the nursing role within the team, few studies have been undertaken. A study of intraprofessional teamwork in district nursing suggests that the goals of teamwork may have primacy over individual patient need and choice. If this is the case in a unidisciplinary team, what is the situation in a multidisciplinary team?

A STUDY OF TEAMS

The remainder of this chapter reports the findings from a study that examined the role of the nurse in rehabilitation work with elderly people. Data were collected from one centre by means of observation and interviews with team members. The findings presented explore the functioning of the multidisciplinary team with particular reference to the role of the nurse.

As we might expect, the consultant was seen as team leader. The following extract from an interview with one consultant physician illustrates the requirement for medical leadership of the team.

> I'm the person who is ultimately responsible for the patients under my care and so I'm the one who has to be responsible for difficult decisions that have to be made, and so from that point of view, I would count myself as the leader.

Another consultant physician concurred with this view.

... Whoever is the consultant is expected by the others to be the leader of the team. I think it would come as a considerable surprise and probably 'shock horror' by the physiotherapist if he or she were expected to lead the team.

It was recognized both by consultant and other staff that decisions made could be challenged.

I think, if you ask them, you will find that the physios, OTs and nursing staff can all quite easily change my decision, and they do. But that's the whole point of having such a meeting, it stops individual members jumping to the wrong conclusions.

While recognizing the ability of staff to challenge consultants' decisions, medical leadership was assumed to be the 'default setting'.

Table 9b.2 illustrates the nature of information sought and given by the multidisciplinary team in case conference situations. Clearly, it is not an exhaustive list of duties that should or could be performed by the respective team members. But the list provides an insight into the compartmentalization of rehabilitation work on the ward. The table demonstrates the wide variety of knowledge nurses were expected to have in contrast to the more specialized knowledge sought from

Table 9b.2 Information giving in the multidisciplinary case conference

Discipline	Information sought
Medical staff	Medical problems, information given by relatives.
Nurses	Frequency of required nursing care, night care, continence, bowel function, state of skin, patients' abilities on the ward, discussion with relatives, patients' questions or views, patients' ability to manage at home
Physiotherapists	Mobility, standing, transferring, walking. Aids required. Chest problems.
Occupational therapists	Feeding capabilities, aids required, dressing capabilities, assessment of daily living activities.
Speech therapist	Communication problems, swallowing problems.
Social workers	Social support at home. Property repairs, pets.

therapists and other team members. Nurses were asked about continence much more often than about any other activity of daily living.

In contrast, the physiotherapist and occupational therapist, social worker and doctors were asked about a specific and narrow range of subjects. This highlights a difference between the nurse and the other multidisciplinary team members, namely that the role of therapists was fairly circumscribed in contrast to the wide range of knowledge that nurses were expected to possess.

It is clear from this small context-specific study and from other literature that the nursing contribution in multidisciplinary meetings is broad rather than deep, and that the nurse's role is that of information giver rather than decision maker. The latter role is ascribed to the medical consultant. A study by Engstrom demonstrated that training nurses to be the chairman or chairwoman of a multidisciplinary clinical team reduced the amount of purely medical communication and increased the attention paid to patients' psychological needs. Engstrom notes: 'if all members of the multidisciplinary clinical team are to consider themselves engaged in the conference, then they must have the possibility to participate through reporting what they themselves know', and 'the physician needs to change his view of the health and illness care file in order to allow significant roles, besides his own, to be featured and valued'.

These observations raise questions about the role of the nurse in the team. In particular, attention must be paid to the needs of nurses who are required to understand, support and continue the work of other team members.

REFERENCES

Evers, H.K. (1981) Tender Loving Care? Patients and Nurses in Geriatric Wards, in *Care of the Ageing* (ed. L.A. Copp), Churchill Livingstone, Edinburgh.

Fairhurst, E. (1981) 'What Do You Do?': Multiple Realities in Occupational Therapy and Rehabilitation, in *Medical Work: Realities and Routines* (eds P. Atkinson and C. Heath), Gower, Farnborough.

Royal College of Nursing/British Geriatric Society/Royal College of Psychiatrists (1987) *Improving Care of Elderly People in Hospital*, Royal College of Nursing, London.

Waters, K.R. (1991) The role of the nurse in the rehabilitation of elderly people in hospital. PhD thesis, University of Manchester.

Webb, A.L. and Hobdell, M. (1980) Co-ordination and Teamwork in the Health and Personal Social Services, in *Teamwork in the Personal Services and Health Care* (eds S. Lonsdale, A.L. Webb and T.L. Briggs), Croom Helm, London.

Occupational therapists 9c

Christine A. Graham

EDITORS' INTRODUCTION

The preceeding chapter demonstrates that nursing input to the multidisciplinary team is adaptable and multifunctional. Occupational therapists have a key role in enhancing and optimizing function following injury or loss. This chapter reviews the various roles of the occupational therapist and the wide-ranging contributions he/she makes to the multidisciplinary team.

Key topics
- Definition and philosophy
- Principal activities
- Developments
- Primary care role
- Future prospects

DEFINITION AND PHILOSOPHY

The present role of occupational therapy within the multidisciplinary team may be complex and, of course, differs from team to team and case to case. This is due in part to the interplay within the team and within occupational therapy. In general, the occupational therapist routinely acts as clinician, adviser, educator and manager.

Occupational therapy has been defined (COT, 1990) as the treatment of people with physical and psychiatric illness or disability through specific selected occupation for the purpose of enabling individuals to reach their maximum level of function and independence in all aspects of life. The occupational therapist assesses the physical, psychological and social functions of the individual, identifies areas of dysfunction, and involves the individual in a structured programme of activity to overcome disability. The activities selected relate to the consumer's personal, social, cultural and economic needs, and reflect the environmental factors that govern his/her lifestyle (COT, 1990).

The philosophy of occupational therapy in this context is to promote and restore health and well-being in people of all

Quality Care for Elderly People. Edited by Peter P. Mayer, Edward J. Dickinson and Martin Sandler. Published in 1997 by Chapman & Hall, London. ISBN 0 412 61830 3

ages through using problem solving and purposeful occupation. Purposeful occupation denotes the meaningful use of various activities, occupations and life roles which can enable people to function purposefully in daily life.

PRINCIPAL ACTIVITIES

Prevention of deterioration or avoidance of predictable problems may be achieved by advice and instruction, or by practicing appropriate skills. Simple examples include joint protection advice for patients with arthritis, transferring to/ from commodes. Assessment of personal and environmental needs indicates adjustment of lifestyle and environment, and provision of equipment or adaptations, where necessary. Such an assessment would commonly include home visiting to assess for toilet and bathing equipment, seating, access into and around the home. In more complex situations adapting the environment for wheelchair use might be required.

Occupational therapy input into rehabilitation requires realistic assessment of function and need, with clear understanding of the prognosis for recovery. Learning of new techniques and skills to promote personal independence are based on mutually agreed goals. Simple examples include basic activities of daily living, such as dressing, cooking, and toileting, as well as more complex skills such as shopping and advice on coping with memory problems or managing challenging behaviour.

Equipment used according to the prescription of the therapist can promote independence. Assessment and advice on the selection of suitable equipment to meet specific individual needs can enhance the quality of life, for example, special cutlery, wheelchair and a hoist for manual handling. Instruction and training in the use of the equipment by the individual or carer(s) is of key importance. However the greatest skill may be required in determining whether, and if so, when, to provide equipment as there may be occasions when it could be counterproductive to the whole rehabilitation process. Most therapists have an anecdote about a patient with good potential to achieve independence, whose overprotective family didn't allow time for the new skills to be practised, provided too much help or inappropriate equipment and compromised the rehabilitative efforts.

Advice on the constructive and creative use of leisure time with ideas for hobbies and social activites can provide therapeutic benefits. This may include individually created activity programmes, and recommendations about the level and type of activity appropriate to the individual's mental, physical and communication capabilities. Advice on specially designed leisure resources might include large print song books or large scale table games.

Occupational therapists have complex advisory and educational roles. Advice to the client and their carer(s) may facilitate enhancement of that individual's independence and quality of life. Advice to other groups may have a wider impact. Advice to other health care workers or to the general public regarding functional assessment and adaptation to lifestyle and environment also has the effect of heightening awareness of occupational therapy and rehabilitation in general. Advice, training and education for home care owners, managers and staff may promote continuing activity (e.g.

Box 9c.1   Range of occupational therapy inputs to older people

Hospital

- Activities of daily living assessments
- Dressing, feeding
- Kitchen assessment
- Assessment of function and remedial treatments
- Home visits
- Activity groups

Primary care/community care

- Joint protection training
- Activities of daily living assessment/treatment
- Assessment of complex needs
- Height of seating, toilet, bed
- Access/egress bath/shower
- Up/down stairs including handrail, stairlift
- Access house, garden, rooms
- Dressing, feeding
- Household – cooking, shopping, laundry, cleaning

Private sector

- Assessments for private nursing homes
- Environment enrichment
- Activity programmes

group work skills and activity programmes), help with management of challenging behaviour (e.g. aggression, confusion), and increase disability awareness (e.g. stroke or dementia).

Thus, occupational therapists may have a wide range of inputs into the care of elderly people (Box 9c.1). The main benefit of occupational therapy is enhancing the quality of life by:

- Restoring skills lost through accident or illness
- Maintaining individuals in their own homes thus delaying/ preventing admission to hospital/residential care
- Facilitating earlier safer discharge from hospital
- Providing support in the community
- Helping to support carers.

This is illustrated in the following example which shows the wide range, of factors that are relevant.

Victoria, British Columbia is highly densley populated with 'seniors'. Quality of life is an expectation and apartments for over 55s are available and include a balcony for air, living area, kitchen for cooking, bathroom, bedroom, all on one level. They are designed with room for walking equipment, an intercom to the warden and a washroom on the ground floor for laundry.

In the area quality of life is catered for by 'walkways' suitable for electric wheelchairs, around the park and along the road to the ocean front, and low floor buses to make getting on easier. There are 'senior' discounts on buses, cheaper rates in restaurants and coffee bars, and entry to popular attractions is at substantially reduced rates.

The total environment is user friendly to people who need to sit at regular intervals, there is level access to shops and shopping malls with covered entry protected from the elements, are popular. Ramp access is aesthetically built into the design of buildings.

In England shop-mobility schemes provide access around shopping areas and there are opportunities to try out vehicles in a realistic setting.

DEVELOPMENTS

Many of the current initiatives have been catalyzed by the Community Care Act, 1990. A variety of services have developed or been enhanced as part of the thrust to reduce the

---

Box 9c.2 Initiatives: what is happening now?

Current developments and issues facing occupational therapists working with elderly people mostly relate to the introduction of the Community Care Act, 1990.

* Hospital/social services seamless care with a massive increase in community-based working; hospital-based occupational therapists going out into the community more.
* Serial home visiting during admission (Shah, 1994).
* Post-discharge follow-up.
* Direct GP referrals; preadmission community visits, e.g. orthopaedic waiting lists, rehabilitation admissions.
* Accident and emergency occupational therapy services (Angier, 1995).
* Hospital at home schemes.
* Primary care occupational therapists attached to GP practices, carrying out 'over-75s' screening checks.
* Residential and nursing homes.
* Housing associations, access and environmental advice.
* Social services waiting lists, interventions by occupational therapists in private practice.

---

requirement for residential care (Box 9c.2). Simultaneously, the length of stays in hospital has been reduced by earlier discharge. The consequence has been a dramatic increase in workload for hospital occupational therapists (especially due to an increases in home visiting). The workload for community-based occupational therapists has risen even more dramatically and is paralleled by the increased dependency of individuals in the community. Consequently, community staffing is beginning to increase, and hospital-based occupational therapy staff are spending more time working in the community, largely performing more home visits sometimes on a serial basis. Post discharge follow up visits are also occurring more frequently, and referrals are being made directly by GPs, and in some cases primary care occupational therapists attached to GP practices carry out the 'over 75s' screening.

Occupational therapists are involved in the various hospital at home schemes. Routine assessments before elective admission, e.g. for orthopaedic surgery, may limit the length of stay in hospital. Input by occupational therapists in the accident and emergency department may reduce admissions and lead to safer discharges following minor trauma (Angier, 1995). There is scope for further development of these roles as rehabilitative services become progressively more community-based.

There is a close working relationship between hospital-based and community-based occupational therapists, although they are employed by different authorities, they usually share responsibility in the resettlement of people at home after hospital care. This ensures continuity in the discharge process and ongoing rehabilitation.

PRIMARY CARE ROLE

The overall aim of the service offered by occupational therapists in primary care is to maintain clients in their own homes and maximize their level of independence. The service offered will include the assessment of individual function in the activities of daily living (ADL). These include washing, dressing, bathing, transfers, cooking and evaluation of the need for provision of equipment and adaptations. This may lead to a planned treatment programme to achieve maximum independence, including teaching new techniques to achieve independence by maximizing abilities, minimizing handicaps, and training carers. This aims to prevent hospital admission by early identification of problems, and by planning prompt treatment and/or therapy within the home, day hospital or as a hospital out-patient. Throughout, there is an emphasis

---

Box 9c.3   Examples of typical patients

- Those with newly diagnosed rheumatoid arthritis
- New minor cerebrovascular accidents
- Those with sudden deterioration or inability to manage, e.g. Parkinson's disease, osteoarthritis
- Those with loss of confidence following a fall
- Those with chronic pain who are unable to tolerate analgesia, e.g. chronic knee/back pain

Box 9c.4   Skills and functions of occupational therapists

Core skills

- Use of purposeful activity and meaningful occupation as therapeutic tools in the promotion of health and well-being.
- Ability to enable people to explore, achieve and maintain balance in the daily living tasks and roles of personal and domestic care, leisure and productivity.
- Ability to assess the effect of, and then to manipulate, physical and psychosocial environments to maximize function and social integration.
- Ability to analyse, select and apply occupations as specific therapeutic media to treat people who are experiencing dysfunction in daily living tasks, interactions and occupational roles.

Aims

- To enable people to maximize their physical, emotional, cognitive, social and functional potential.
- To anticipate and prevent the effects of disability and dysfunction through education and therapeutic intervention in a functional context.
- To enable people to achieve a meaningful lifestyle by preparing for, or returning to, work, or the development of the quality use of time through leisure, education, training and opportunities for voluntary work.
- To provide professional advocacy for people on access and equal opportunities matters.
- To provide practical advice and support for the families and carers of people with disabilities.

Approach

- Ability to change, adapt and modify practices according to the needs of people with disabilities and their environment.
- Partnerships with others to facilitate development of services for people with disabilities.
- Ability to influence social policy and legislation relating to impairment, disability, handicap and economic self-sufficiency.

on counselling, supporting and advising clients and carers. These approaches are applicable in a wide range of situations, and Box 9c.3 lists patients typical of those who might be referred.

FUTURE PROSPECTS

The future prospects of occupational therapy depend on the core skills, objectives and approach of the profession (Box 9c.4).

These features of occupational therapy reflect its central values and belief that people with disabilities are valued as people with physical, emotional, intellectual, social and spiritual needs. Occupational therapists use their core skills to enable and empower people to make choices and to achieve a personally acceptable lifestyle, with the goal of maximizing health and function. This way of working fits well with service developments especially the focus on consumer needs.

In recent years there has been an increase in the number of occupational therapists undertaking work for, or in liaison with, GPs as part of the primary care service. This is probably occurring because the philosophies of occupational therapy and general practice are close. Given the renewed emphasis on community-based health care, appropriate outcomes and needs-based service, the future prospects for occupational therapy look bright.

REFERENCES

Angier, C. (1995) Outcomes of Occupational Therapy. *British Journal of Occupational Therapy*, Vol 58 Feb 1995, 69.

College of Occupational Therapists SPP 140, (1990) *Occupational Therapy Definitions*, COT, London.

National Health Service and Community Care Act 1990, HMSO, London.

Shah, M. (1994) Graduated home visiting programme for the elderly at Wembley Community Hospital. Arjo/Therapy Weekly National Therapy Award.

FURTHER READING

Publications of the College of Occupational Therapists, 6-8 Marshalsea Road, Southwark, London SE1 1HL

Animals in Occupational Therapy Practice	SPP 130, 1990
Audit	SPP 180, 1991
Consent for Occupational Therapy	SPP 195, 1993
Data Protection Act	SPP 155, 1990
OT Services for clients with Learning Disabilities	SPP 115A, 1995
Home Visiting with Hospital In-Patients	SPP 170, 1990
Occupational Therapy Definitions	SPP 140, 1990
OT in Private Practice	SPP 100A, 1994
OT Services for Consumers with Physical Disabilities	SPP 105B, 1995
OT Services in Mental Health	SPP 110A, 1995
Setting up a Quality Assurance Programme	SPP 175, 1991
Statement on OT Referral	SPP 125A, 1994
Therapeutic Intervention by Occupational Therapists with Consumers in their own Homes	SPP 200, 1993
Core Skills and A Conceptual Framework for Practice – A Position Statement	087
Gardening with Disability	011
How OT Helps Stroke Patients	061
OT in Private/Voluntary Sector Residential and Nursing Homes	015

Physiotherapists 9d

Pennie Roberts and
Carole Brown

EDITORS' INTRODUCTION

The therapist contributes to the well-being of individuals by optimizing their quality of life. Improvement in movement is the domain of the physiotherapist and treatment often requires attention to balance, perception and sensory deficits. This chapter provides a brief description of the roles and specialist skills of the physiotherapist and describes examples of successful multidisciplinary teamwork.

Key topics
- Aims and activities
- New models
- Key principles
- Future developments

AIMS AND ACTIVITIES

Physiotherapy is a health care profession that emphasizes the use of physical approaches in the prevention and treatment of disease and disability.

Chartered physiotherapists are consulted in relation to the physical problems of patients, in particular those associated with neuromuscular, musculoskeletal, cardiovascular and respiratory systems, and also the prevention of problems relating to these (CSLT/COT/CSP, 1993). Box 9d.1 lists some of the conditions that benefit from physiotherapy treatment.

The aim of physiotherapy is to improve mobility, psychological well-being and communication skills, thus enabling individuals to optimize their functional ability.

Functional problems may be due to physical or psychological causes. Physiotherapists use physical techniques and modalities to treat these and break the cycle of loss of function, depression and decreased function, however it may have started. The specialist skills available from the physiotherapy service are shown in Box 9d.2.

Quality Care for Elderly People. Edited by Peter P. Mayer, Edward J. Dickinson and Martin Sandler. Published in 1997 by Chapman & Hall, London. ISBN 0 412 61830 3

Box 9d.1 Some of the conditions that benefit from physiotherapy treatment

- Mobility problems
- Strains
- Neck and back problems
- Sports injuries
- Circulatory problems
- Amputees
- Strokes
- Multiple sclerosis
- Rheumatoid and osteoarthritis

NEW MODELS

Physiotherapy has always been able to respond flexibly to new challenges. Different models of working practice have evolved depending on the demands of the situation. Physiotherapists make good team players (Table 9d.1) and can demonstrate their adaptability and responsiveness as structures and organizations change. This is shown in the case of the Derbyshire Dales Rehabilitation Team (Case study 9d.1).

Case study 9d.1 Derbyshire Dales Rehabilitation Team
Throughout 1993 and 1994, the therapy professions – occupational therapy, physiotherapy, chiropody and speech and language therapy – have concentrated on creating a

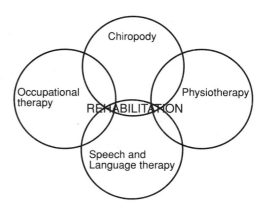

team to provide a co-ordinated rehabilitation service rather than separate services. They have developed their team

Table 9d.1   Examples of teams that include physiotherapists

Type of service	Location
Inpatients	Across all hospital directorates (obstetrics and gynaecology, surgical, medical, care of elderly people, neurology, psychiatry, intensive and coronary care, orthopaedics)
Outpatients	In hospital departments, GP clinics and private practice
Day units	
Biomechanic and appliance clinics	
Continence clinics	
Ante- and Postnatal care	
Community-based service	Own home, residential homes, nursing homes, health centres, schools, child development centres, learning disability specialty teams, primary health care teams

---

Box 9d.2   Specialist skills available from the physiotherapy service

- Elderly rehabilitation
- Acupuncture
- Continence promotion
- Facial palsy treatment
- Varicose ulcers treatment
- Relaxation techniques
- Pressure care
- Gait analysis
- Pain control
- Education in moving and handling
- Back school

---

concept with its obvious benefits to patient care while maintaining their individual professional identity.

Many factors have helped to created better team working, not the least of which is a joint communication programme, a joint in-service training programme and a joint quality assurance programme.

In-service training is being provided for occupational therapy and physiotherapy assistants to create therapy assistants. This is being achieved by increasing the skills of both occupational therapy and physiotherapy assistants so they become support workers for both services.

Many joint initiatives have arisen throughout 1993 and 1994, including the biomechanics assessment and appliance clinic, which won the NHS Quality Award. A more co-ordinated approach has been created through the integration of the three services.

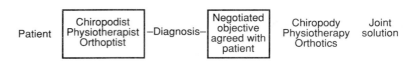

The Derbyshire Dales Rehabilitation Team has been extremely successful in developing collaborative working – an emphasis being on providing one-stop services to meet the needs of local people.

Case study 9d.2   Disability Resource Team

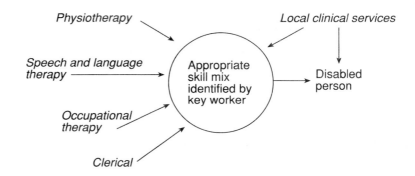

The Disability Resource Team

This team works with physically disabled people and their carers to prevent inappropriate hospital admission, promote independent living, and support the provision of community care. Recruited initially for their specific therapy skills individual team members provide an integrated service, calling on the skills of their colleagues in the team and from elsewhere as appropriate. Physiotherapy skills are fed into the process both by the team member and also by locally managed mainstream physiotherapists. These principles are highly applicable to the care of older people and are illustrated in the figure above.

The input of physiotherapists into multidisciplinary teams is further illustrated by the 'Going for Gold' initiative (Case study 9d.3).

Case study 9d.3   'Going for Gold'

Recognition that physiotherapy input into the prevention, treatment and ongoing management of pressure sores was not always co-ordinated with that of other professionals has led to a series of initiatives. These have been highly successful in combining the skills and knowledge of several groups, including physiotherapists, and dramatically reducing the number of pressure sores.

The project had input from pharmacists, nurses, physiotherapists, disabled people and carers. It aimed to eliminate pressure sores in patients in all sectors and agencies - acute hospital, community services, the private sector, residential and nursing homes, and the district nursing service. The Going for Gold initiative was based on common education, agreed practice and clear outcomes. Its success has demonstrated the effectiveness of team work in dealing with has been an intractable problem in health care provision.

FUTURE DEVELOPMENTS

The future of health care is in community settings. Physiotherapists have the skills necessary to ensure that primary health care teams can work effectively and deliver good quality health care in a rapidly changing environment. The ever increasing demand for physiotherapists means that skills must be used effectively, and this will mean working in a variety of ways. Physiotherapists have always been involved in hands-on clinical practice, assessment and diagnosis, education, advice and consultancy. These roles need to be used to best advantage to ensure the team is complemented and can work as a coherent whole. The profession has developed new skills of management, marketing and manipulation, while retaining its core clinical base of massage, movement, exercise and electrotherapy. The appropriate use of this wide and unique skill base will provide patients with excellent care, and the team, in whatever form, with a rich and varied pool of expertise.

REFERENCE

College of Speech and Language Therapists College of Occupational Therapists and Chartered Society of Physiotherapy (1993) *Promoting Collaborative Practice*, CSLT/COT/CSP, London.

Social workers 9e

Barbara Laing

<table>
<tr><td colspan="2">

EDITORS' INTRODUCTION

The roles of the remedial therapists previously discussed are wider than might initially be appreciated. However, no other individual within the multidisciplinary team is considered as completely holistic as the social worker. In this chapter the responsibilities of the social worker are described and some of the incongruities and anomalies of this role highlighted.

Key topics
- Social workers and society
- The role of the social worker
- Work with carers
- Dilemmas in social work
- Recent developments

</td></tr>
</table>

SOCIAL WORKERS AND SOCIETY

Social workers work predominantly within a psychosocial framework, addressing the fears, worries and practical needs of elderly people. However, many of the issues that social workers wrestle with, particularly financial deprivation, are beyond their control, resting as they do within the social and political construction of poverty and dependency (Phillipson, 1982). The poverty experienced by many elderly people reflects society's lack of investment in the older generation. The consequences directly and drastically affect individuals and their carers in their ability to control and manage their own lifestyles. People with disabilities require increased financial resources in order to meet their needs (Harris, 1972; Walker, 1976; Townsend, 1979), and black and minority ethnic elderly people' are disproportionately represented in low income groups (Blackburn, 1992). The values and principles that underpin social work must therefore be concerned with issues of inequality, discrimination and oppression, and the profession is set within a political and hence, at times, controversial context.

Quality Care for Elderly People. Edited by Peter P. Mayer, Edward J. Dickinson and Martin Sandler. Published in 1997 by Chapman & Hall, London. ISBN 0 412 61830 3

As with medicine, many of the situations facing social workers have no simple or easy answers, and involve long journeys through moral and ethical mazes (Jordan, 1990). The result is a 'damned if they do' and 'damned if they don't' response to some of the more publicized pieces of work. Coupled with accusations of 'political correctness', and severe resourcing problems, it is easy to see why social workers frequently feel isolated and marginalized by other professionals. No discussion of social work would be complete without an acknowledgement of the tensions that exist between this profession and others working within the field of elderly care. However, my own experience is that appreciation of the role of social work in enabling the delivery of high quality care to older people is often expressed at a local, individual practitioner level, while generalized, somewhat sceptical, attitudes to the profession continue.

ROLE OF THE SOCIAL WORKER

It is hard to describe the role of the social worker succinctly, and this demonstrates both its strengths and weaknesses. Social workers share many of the skills and tasks of other professionals – enhancing mental health, providing counselling, welfare benefits and housing advice, providing access to services, support to carers, etc. What is perhaps unique is the fact that social workers are truly holistic in their approach, finding all aspects of the elderly person's psychological and social situation important in their assessment. Social workers aim to work at a pace that enables the elderly person to play a central and active part in the assessment and decision making processes. The timing of their work may therefore be in conflict with the needs of other professionals or organizations. This is thrown into high relief when hospital discharge planning is being undertaken. The pressure to clear beds frequently results in elderly people being 'processed' and their views and wishes not actively addressed (Wilkinson, 1985; Townsend, 1986a; Victor and Vetter, 1988).

Social work does not find itself allied to the 'medical model'. The identification, diagnosis and treatment of pathological conditions holds little in common with the social work approach. Rather, by working in partnership with elderly people, their families and carers, social workers attempt to identify just what it is that needs to be changed or supplied so that people's goals can be achieved. This may seem a somewhat idealistic view of life in later years as, for many professionals and elderly people themselves, aspirations relating to this period of life are generally low (Phillipson, 1982). However, integral to the social worker's role is the need to combat and challenge ageist beliefs that allow such attitudes to continue and result in a patronizing, directional and oppressive approach towards elderly people (Townsend, 1986b). At the heart of excellence within social work is the identification of the needs of the individual, especially when these are in conflict with those of others.

The acknowledgement and negotiation of conflict is where the social worker is able to demonstrate particular skills. This work can be especially challenging when issues of risk are considered. At times, we all take risks and, unless we are likely to cause significant harm to those around us, we are generally free to make our own choices, but expect to live with the consequences. Elderly people frequently find their choices are limited, and while the concerned actions of others may ostensibly be aimed at protecting them, the result is often an infringement of rights based on 'infantilized' notions (Phillipson, 1982). Thus the social worker may well be acting in an advocacy role, negotiating and explaining to others the reasons why the wishes and decisions of the elderly person should be respected, albeit that those decisions place him or her at some – even considerable – risk. Such stances are often adopted in relation to those who have cognitive impairment and whose ability to fully comprehend the significance of their decisions is in doubt. These are perhaps among the most difficult situations facing the social worker, and, indeed, other members of the multidisciplinary team and family. Case study 9e.1 explores this issue further.

Case study 9e.1

The local social worker was asked by a neighbour if he would visit Enid because she was often found to be wearing her nightclothes during the day and was sleeping in a chair. Enid had mild memory problems which had resulted in her leaving her cooker on, and recently there had been a small fire in her kitchen. Enid herself said she was happy living at home, had no problems, but liked it when the Home Carer visited each Wednesday to do some housework and shopping. It transpired that Enid would only allow the Home Carer to assist her in changing her clothes and washing now and again. As a result, Enid appeared unkempt and was somewhat smelly. Enid's sister, appalled at the state she was in, was insisting that she be admitted to a residential home even though this was clearly against Enid's wishes. The social worker spent time with the neighbours and Enid's sister explaining Enid's point of view and the fact that, although there were risks involved, these were comparable with those for many people living in the community. The neighbours accepted this, but her sister was unable to and withdrew, making threats that the social worker would be held accountable if anything happened to Enid.

The social worker has little recourse to the law to provide a framework to support either risk-taking or the assumption of rights over the elderly person – unlike the social worker's access to child care legislation (Age Concern, 1986). Social workers in these circumstances often find themselves working in a legislative vacuum, having to constantly refer back to the issues of self-determination, empowerment and choice that drive their work (Case study 9e.2).

Case study 9e.2
Grace, aged 85, was admitted to hospital with an acute chest infection. While there it became clear that she had severe dementia with poor short-term memory. Although physically able, she was reliant on others for her orientation, personal care and safety.

She lived in an inner city area with her friend Albert. Albert had mental health problems that caused him to be afraid and suspicious of those around him. The front door was barred and he would only talk to visitors through the letterbox. Eventually, the social worker was able to gain his confidence and obtain access to the house. She discovered the house to be in a poor structural and decorative state. Upstairs was the skeleton of a cat that had obviously died some time before, and rats were seen running around. Grace maintained that she wished to return home, but it was clear that she would need a large package of care to sustain her, which Albert was not prepared to accept.

Prior to her admission she had clearly been very unwell for some days, but Albert had seen no reason to go for help, assuming that Grace was tired. Grace appeared to enjoy life in the hospital and made no attempt to leave. However, each time her discharge was discussed she said she wished to return home and it was evident that she had no insight into her situation. After much deliberation, specialist advice and debate, Grace was admitted to a local authority residential home. It was not possible to exercise any statutory powers to confirm this decision, which was based on the unacceptable risk to Grace of her returning home, but was clearly against her stated wishes.

WORK WITH CARERS

Many elderly people rely on formal and informal carers in order to remain within their own homes. Many such carers are themselves elderly, often female, and in poor health (Levin, Sinclair and Gorbach, 1990). For carers, the stress can be enormous, and when this is compounded by long-standing relationship difficulties, the quality of care and the capacity to continue caring is diminished. It may not be until, say, an admission to hospital, that such tensions come to light. Social workers can assist by 'unpicking' the origins of the stress and encouraging elderly people and their carers to acknowledge the reality of their situation.

Many carers are bound by a mixture of feelings, including obligation, guilt and anger, which are frequently hard to express openly (Pitkeathley, 1989). Not only can social workers encourage the expression and sharing of these feelings, but they can offer reassurance that such feelings, although painful, are normal. The elderly person may equally hold a mixture of emotions regarding his or her need to receive care from others, and an opportunity to express feelings, although not changing the reality of the situation, again frequently helps.

Through their knowledge of local and national voluntary organizations, social workers can encourage elderly people and their carers to contact groups and organizations that may provide them with understanding support, help, information and encouragement from others with similar experiences. The comprehensive nature of their work enables social workers to be well-informed about the totality of elderly people's experiences and therefore their needs. Thus, social workers can play a central role as activists in developing community-based services and in promoting collective action by elderly people themselves.

Social workers also act as key holders to many services that enable carers to continue caring and elderly people to remain at home. Most local authorities provide a range of home (help) care, day and respite care together with services designed to meet the particular needs of black and minority ethnic people. The development of both health and social services for black and minority ethnic people is generally accepted as an area in need of expansion: most social workers would agree that the choices for black people, their families and carers are extremely limited (Norman, 1985), as Case study 9e.3 illustrates.

Case study 9e.3
Yu Lee had immigrated to the UK three years before having a severe stroke. She had come from Hong Kong to live with her son and daughter-in-law, but the level of care she needed meant that they were unable to have her home again. It was agreed that Yu would go to a nursing home, but the family was unable to find one that had other members of the Chinese community for Yu to converse with. She was therefore admitted to a home near the family, so that she could be visited regularly, but whose elderly residents were white Europeans. The social worker made arrangements for Yu to attend a Chinese Day Centre across the city so that she could have the company of those who shared her culture and language. Although this went some way to meeting her needs, Yu (unlike white elderly people) had not had any choice of homes that would address her basic need for communication.

DILEMMAS IN SOCIAL WORK

Phillipson (1982) argues that social workers uphold systems that disadvantage those in need, by using techniques of 'coercion and passivity', and that this results in the lowering of expectations of elderly people themselves. However, social workers are increasingly facing a dichotomy. Given the level of poverty experienced by many elderly people, the knowledge and expertise that many social workers hold in relationship to welfare rights is important in ensuring that incomes are maximized through timely and appropriate applications for benefits. The need to maximize income is even more crucial when the social worker's role as a means tester is considered. Services increasingly attract charges, and social workers are required to complete not only needs-based assessments, but also financial assessments which detail the service users' liability to pay.

Within Social Services Department there is a very live debate on the achievement of a balance between the provision of community-based care and residential care. Some elderly people actively choose to live in residential and nursing home facilities, perhaps because of fears of isolation and vulnerability. For others, though, the choice is not quite so positive. It is often not possible for individuals requiring even a moderate amount of personal care to remain within their own homes because of limitations in domiciliary care services (Case study 9e.4), while access to residential care is available.

Case study 9e.4
Lucy made a good recovery from the amputation of her leg, and was reasonably mobile using her Zimmer frame. She lived alone, but had the support of neighbours and a niece who visited once a week to do the shopping. Lucy needed some assistance in washing and dressing and negotiating the three steps from her bedroom to her sitting room. Whilst home care was available each weekday to help with these activities, there was no care at weekends. Lucy rejected the option of remaining in the one room all day, and also disliked being more dependent on her neighbours. She was unable to afford the cost of private care over the weekend and therefore opted for residential care.

RECENT DEVELOPMENTS

For some elderly people, the supply and fitting of specialized aids and adaptations may prove to be the key to remaining within their own homes. In addition, social service departments do offer a variety of care that is increasingly designed to meet the particular needs of individual elderly people and their carers. For some it is the nights that are most problematic, when the elderly person does not wish to, or cannot, sleep and is waking others or wandering outside. Some areas have developed 24-hour day care to offer support to carers and to enable elderly people to receive the care and attention they require at a time when many other services are not available. Respite care is also being used increasingly to support both elderly people and their carers in remaining at home for the majority of the time.

The changes in health care, especially the move towards day surgery and the shorter length of inpatient stay, have highlighted the need to ensure a high quality of discharge planning and post-discharge support. The role of the hospital social work team is crucial in informing and empowering older people and their carers to access services (McLeod, 1994). There is a need to continue to develop a rapid response and flexible home care service. In many cases there has been a transformation in the home care service, shifting it from a housework service to one that offers personal care to those with a high level of need. For many social services departments, the dialogue and development of innovative projects with health purchasers and providers is of high priority. However, the fragmentation of health care provision makes joint working complex in the extreme.

There is little doubt that social workers play an important part in enabling and assisting elderly people and their carers to maximize their potential. Central to their role must be the confrontation of discrimination which disempowers and disables elderly people and their carers, limiting their control and choices. Most social workers remain frustrated by the lack of adequate welfare provision for elderly people, and are committed to offering and delivering a service that is appropriate and sensitive to their needs. Their role is complex, difficult and challenging, as are the issues they are addressing.

REFERENCES

Age Concern (1986) *The Law and Vulnerable People*, Age Concern England, London.

Blackburn, C. (1992) *Improving Health and Welfare Work with Families in Poverty*, Open University Press, Milton Keynes.

Harris, A.I. (1972) *Income and Entitlement to Supplementary Benefit of Impaired People in Great Britain*, HMSO, London.

Jordan, B. (1992) *Social Work in an Unjust Society*, Harvester Wheatsheaf, Hemel Hempstead.

Levin, E., Sinclair, I. and Gorbach, P. (1990) *Families, Services and Confusion in Old Age*, National Institute for Social Work Research Unit, Avebury, Aldershot.

McLeod, E. (1995) The strategic importance of hospital social work. *Social Work and Social Science Review,* vol VI (1) pp. 19–32.

Norman, A.J. (1985) *Triple Jeopardy: Growing Old in a Second Homeland*, Centre for Policy on Ageing, London.

Phillipson, C. (1982) *Capitalism and the Construction of Old Age*, Macmillan, London.

Pitkeathley, J. (1989) *Daughters Who Care: Daughters Caring for Mothers at Home*, Routledge, London.

Townsend, A. (1986a) *Family Caregivers' Perspectives on Institutional Decision Making*, University of Tennessee.

Townsend, P. (1979) *Poverty in the United Kingdom*, Pelican, Harmondsworth.

Townsend, P. (1986b) Ageism and Social Policy, in *Ageing and Social Policy: A Critical Assessment* (eds C. Phillipson and A. Walker), Gower, Aldershot.

Victor, C.R. and Vetter, N.J. (1988) Preparing the elderly for discharge from hospital: a neglected aspect of patient care? *Age and Ageing*, **17**, 155–63.

Walker, A. (1976) *Living Standards in Crisis*, Disability Alliance, London.

FURTHER READING

Mcleod (1994) *Patients in Interprofessional Practice*, Edward Arnold, London.

Teamwork 10

Ann Hunter

<table>
<tr><td>

EDITORS' INTRODUCTION

The previous sections have defined the role of a number of different core clinical professionals in the elderly services' multidisciplinary team. Many other professional disciplines contribute on an 'as required' basis, such as speech therapy, dietetics, psychology, chiropody and a variety of services such as dental, vision and hearing. Therefore to provide good quality care excellent co-ordination of both a full- and part-time team is needed.

This chapter looks at the elements of good and poor team practice. The types of teams that exist are described as well as the roles and functions of members of the team, functions that improve and decrease the effectiveness of the elements of leadership, and the components of successful leadership, with guidance on building successful health care teams.

</td><td>

Key topics
- Definition
- Team roles
- Team dynamics
- Barriers to effective teams
- Successful teams

</td></tr>
</table>

DEFINITION

Teams do not happen – they require strong leadership, clear role definitions and common objectives. Many factors may stop professionals changing from a group to a team and need to be recognized and tackled.

In health care, the term 'team' is widely used to describe people working together in the same area, hopefully towards the same goal. To the man or woman in the street, the term usually applies to sport, where one team needs to compete against another to function in that role. Competition is essential to the functioning of teams in sports, and it may bring out the best or the worst in a team, often depending on whether it is winning or losing. It is assumed that each team has a captain, a coach and a manager. Everyone understands the

Quality Care for Elderly People. Edited by Peter P. Mayer, Edward J. Dickinson and Martin Sandler. Published in 1997 by Chapman & Hall, London. ISBN 0 412 61830 3

function of each team member. The rules of the game are well established and, indeed, available in print. Another important point is the reward of winning – not only the glory but the financial prize, too. The immediate and most obvious difference between a sports team and a health care one is of motivating factors. Even in sport, teams do not function well if the players are of poor quality and have a poor manager.

Katzenbach and Smith (1993) describe the team as 'a small number of people with complementary skills who are committed to a common purpose, set of performance goals, and approach for which they hold themselves mutually accountable'.

This description from the business world also applies to health care teams. Clear distinctions are drawn on the differences between groups and teams (Table 10.1).

Teams have been promoted as the most effective way of producing high quality health care for elderly people. The Cumberlege Report (1986) and the Government's White Paper *Promoting Better Health* (Department of Health, 1987) both advocated the use of multiprofessional teams. Quality standards in purchasers' contracts for provider units often include multidisciplinary assessment and evidence of team work as essential standards of care. The literature abounds with examples of teamwork, but little evidence exists of effective teams improving health care. A study on complementary medicine by Reason (1991), however, describes the power struggle within the group, not only over the group purpose but also over the group philosophy. Comments and complaints are constantly heard about poor communication and fragmented services.

Table 10.1 Not all groups are teams: how to tell the difference

Working group	*Team*
• Strong clearly focused leader	• Shared leadership roles
• Individual accountability	• Individual and mutual accountability
• The group's purpose is the same as the broader organizational mission	• Specific team purpose that the team itself delivers
• Individual work-products	• Collective work-products
• Runs efficient meetings	• Encourages open-ended discussion and active problem-solving meetings
• Measures its effectiveness indirectly by its influence on others (e.g. financial performance of the business)	• Measures performance directly by assessing collective work-products
• Discusses, decides and delegates	• Discusses, decides and does real work together

Teams can be both uniprofessional and multiprofessional. District nurses, health visitors and practice nurses working in the community may see themselves as the community nursing team. The other professional groups see themselves as the multidisciplinary team. Uniprofessional teams often cut across the authority of multiprofessional teams, making accountability and leadership key issues.

Ovretveit (1993) describes the multidisciplinary team in the community as 'a group of practitioners with different professional training (multidisciplinary), employed by more than one agency (multiagency), who meet regularly to co-ordinate their work providing services to one or more clients in a defined area'.

Teams working in acute hospital settings also fit this framework. For example, the liaison sister for the elderly care team may be based in the accident and emergency department, but employed by the community trust. The occupational therapist who deals with resettlement into the community may be employed by social services. Although the author has encountered community-based teams for elderly people with mental health problems, most services for elderly people are still hospital-based.

Team type
• Uniprofessional
• Multiprofessional
• The former may cut across the latter

Types of team

Ovretveit (1993) describes three types of team:

- client teams
- network teams
- formal teams.

A **client** team consists of all the people involved in any one part of the client's episode of care. A team from a provider unit led by a care manager is an example of this type of team. Although a client could have a different team and a different care manager for each stage of the health care process, this lack of continuity would lead to confusion. The main working relationship in these teams is between the care manager and each individual client.

A **network** team is a voluntary grouping of health care workers who do not necessarily subscribe to the same values or objectives and may be accountable to different people. There is no formal leader and the members usually belong to and identify with another team.

A **formal** team is a permanent group of people dealing with the same client group in the same area, e.g. the day hospital or the assessment unit. Ovretveit found that permanent teams differed in three main ways:

- the level of integration of team members
- the composition of the team and how it is managed
- how the patient/client process of care is dealt with over time.

TEAM ROLES

Health care teams
- Developed by default
- Common goal
- Functional roles

In health care, teams tend to be developed by default rather than specially selected. In other words, the various professional groups represented are working towards a common goal in a special area of health care that may relate to a specific client or diagnostic group. Each person has a professional function within the team that is assumed from the other team members' knowledge of that profession. When new teams are formed, each member is usually picked for his/her function rather than his/her team role.

Although team members may be excellent in their professional role, they may be unclear about their team role. Perhaps because of this, Belbin's concept of team roles (1981) has found much favour in the health sector. This work was based on research at Henley in the 1970s. From psychometric testing eight team types were identified. Certain people assumed certain roles within the team, with the pattern of role balance affecting the success of the team.

Models for team roles
- Belbin
- Team management index
- Spencer and pruss

When, a decade later, Belbin (1993) discusses the further evolution of team roles, the specialist has been added as the role of the professional expert (Table 10.2). This acknowledges individuals who have a strong preference to become more specialized and expert in a certain area. Furthermore, two roles had had a name change because of the status implications that were associated with their initial role: chairman, which inferred a hierarchical structure, was changed to co-ordinator; and company worker was changed to implementer for the same reason.

The Belbin model has been extremely useful in enabling teams to identify their strengths and weaknesses. Dr Belbin has developed a computer-based assessment system called Interplace, which integrates self-reporting with observer assessments. This should help to overcome the problem of the self-reporting questionnaire being limited to how self-aware the individual is.

Table 10.2 The nine team roles

Roles	Descriptions – team-role contribution	Allowable weaknesses
Plant	Creative, imaginative, unorthodox; solves difficult problems	Ignores details; too preoccupied to communicate effectively
Resource investigator	Extrovert, enthusiastic, communicative; explores opportunities; develops contacts	Overoptimistic; loses interest once initial enthusiasm has passed
Co-ordinator	Mature, confident, a good chairperson; clarifies goals, promotes decision making, delegates well	Can be seen as manipulative; delegates personal work
Shaper	Challenging, dynamic, thrives on pressure; has the drive and courage to overcome obstacles	Can provoke others; hurts people's feelings
Monitor evaluator	Sober, strategic and discerning; sees all options; judges accurately	Lacks drive and ability to inspire others; overly critical
Teamworker	Co-operative, mild, perceptive and diplomatic; listens, builds, averts friction, calms the waters	Indecisive in crunch situations; can be easily influenced
Implementer	Disciplined, reliable, conservative and efficient; turns ideas into practical actions	Somewhat inflexible; slow to respond to new possibilities
Completer	Painstaking, conscientious, anxious; searches out errors and omissions; delivers on time	Inclined to worry unduly; reluctant to delegate; can be a nit-picker
Specialist	Single-minded, self-starting, dedicated; provides knowledge and skills in rare supply	Contributes on only a narrow front; dwells on technicalities; overlooks the 'big picture'

Strength of contribution in any one of the roles is commonly associated with particular weaknesses. These are called allowable weaknesses. Executives are seldom strong in all nine team roles.

Magerison and McCann (1987) developed a Team Management Index (TMI) questionnaire, based on Jung's introversion/extroversion theory, that identifies people's work preferences. In their extensive research they focused on four main areas:

• how people prefer to relate to each other
• how people prefer to gain or use information

• how people prefer to make decisions
• how people prefer to organize themselves and others.

The scores from the TMI are depicted on the Team Management Wheel (Figure 10.1), showing one sector as the main preference and another two as 'back-up' roles. This method can be used to help with team selection and development. I have found it helpful in balancing team membership: new members are less likely to be based on my own image; and it highlights not only the individual strengths of each team member, but also the skill gaps in the team.

Spencer and Pruss (1992) are critical of the 'blurring' of definitions between team roles and personality types and believe that the complexities of team dynamics require the definitions to be separated. They then identify 10 functional roles.

• The **visionary** has the overall vision of the team mission as well as a perspective of where that mission fits into the wider organizational objectives.
• The **pragmatist** reminds the visionary of the practical implications and realities, but also attempts to make the impossible possible, by suggesting alternatives.

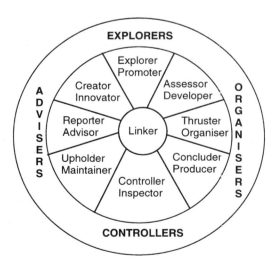

Figure 10.1   Team management wheel.

- The **explorer** seeks information, material and support from outside the team environment, building bridges between the team and other teams.
- The **challenger** requests that the team review its own definition of objectives and progress, and challenges suggestions and proposals from the team members.
- The **referee** takes as near an independent view of team progress as possible.
- The **peacemaker** sees that fair play is done and harmonizes between conflicting views.
- The **beaver** does all the work!
- The **coach** boosts morale and gives positive re-enforcement.
- The **librarian** records team activities and can give team members feedback on past actions.
- The **confessor** provides a shoulder to cry on and maintains confidentiality.

Spencer and Pruss also make the important point that people function differently in different teams. The functions are separated from personality as far as possible. The role of the team leader in this situation is to recognize which people in that particular situation exhibit the particular balance of characteristics needed to take on the particular roles in question. This model may rest well within the health care framework when the same people are members of different teams.

TEAM DYNAMICS

Tuckman (1965) defined four stages of team development – forming, storming, norming and performing – which describe the behaviours and structure of the group.

> **Stages of team development**
> - Forming
> - Storming
> - Norming
> - Performing

Forming

In this stage group members are coming to terms with how they might deal with their task and are dependent on the leader. The main objective is clarification of team goals and accepting the behaviours and actions of the other members of the group.

Storming

In the second stage, conflict emerges in the group from role competitiveness and defensiveness. The group resolves the conflict and concentrates on the task in hand.

Norming

Now the group is more accepting of each other's differences and each individual is feeling part of the team, creating new parameters for group behaviour and becoming more cohesive.

Performing

At the final stage, the team members are working towards achieving the common goal of the group. By now the roles are more flexible within the group and the leadership role is shared among the group members.

This model has been adapted and developed by others and indeed expanded by the original author (Tuckman and Jensen, 1977) to include adjouring. Anderson (1993), in her literature review of the team process, found common ground in the various models that have been developed in the 1980s and 1990s.

Movement from one stage to the next depends on achieving the tasks and goals of the previous stage. Interpersonal concerns have also to be resolved before moving on to the next stage. Some teams fluctuate between stages if there are personnel or task changes. The team experiences highs and lows, and team building activities help to move the team more quickly through the various stages.

The Hawthorn studies of the 1920s and 1930s investigated the effect of the working environment on productivity. He found that the stronger the group identity and the more constructive the interest of the leader/manager, the more effective the group.

The development of organizational analysis theory in the 1960s by Likert and McGregor led to the accepted characteristics of the effective work group. Most modern writers agree with these attributes.

- Roles – skilled in the various roles.
- Time – this is required to establish good working relationships.

- Loyalty to the team.
- Trust in each other.
- The values and goals of the team reflect the values and goals of the team members.
- Decision making and problem solving occurs in a supportive atmosphere.
- The leader possesses the appropriate skills for that role (Dyer, 1977).

BARRIERS TO EFFECTIVE TEAMS

Accountability

Within the health sector the hierarchical structure mitigates against team working and the provision of comprehensive health care. Navarro (1987) suggests that while most of the population will need some kind of health care at some time in their lives, health teams tend to focus on diagnosis and are led by doctors who follow a 'cure' philosophy. They are often widely accepted as the acknowledged experts and are assumed to be in charge of the other health professionals. In elderly care, where medical and social problems merge and a more holistic concept is prevalent, the potential for conflict is always there.

Decreasing effectiveness
• Hierachy
• Dual accountability
• Unclear professional autonomy

The professions allied to medicine have clung to a function-led management structure that cuts across teams operating around a specialist clinical area or within the primary care or the community. In directorate structures these professions often loose their professional leader which, instead of promoting better team working, often leaves them feeling very vulnerable. The role of this leader was both operational, to manage the service efficiently and effectively, and professional, to develop and maintain the clinical professional skills. Clinical teams functioning in health care are further complicated by management structures cutting across the team function. Team members have accountability to a professional head as well as to the leader of the team.

Dual accountability is more acceptable in social services where they have clear definitions about who does what. Nurses, who were used to a hierarchical structure, often appear to have an ill-defined accountability and management role.

The issue of accountability is further complicated by a lack of clarity on professional autonomy. Most of the professions allied to medicine are accountable to themselves for their own professional practice. The medical profession has, in the main, accepted this, but moving from a situation when work was prescribed by doctors to make their own clinical decisions had been difficult for some professions, in particular nurses, partly because of clinical judgement and clinical freedom. The professional bodies may need to provide stronger leadership in professional issues allowing the management function to occur at a more local level.

Common sense would suggest that large teams function less well than small teams (eight members and fewer) because the more people involved in communication the more difficult it is. Chaudhry-Lawton *et al.* (1992) have found that teams of more than 10 people or fewer than three function least well. They cite a model of subteams or cells in industry which seemed very effective.

When discussing primary health care and community teams, Pritchard (1995) suggests that large teams can communicate on a one to one basis or the team could split into firms, still retaining the same co-ordinator. He found this system to work successfully in Iceland and Sweden. In some community settings if each member of each profession wishes to be included in the team it is too large. The 'small is beautiful' concept often prevails with less potential conflict being evident with fewer people.

Teams often need to familiarize themselves with the environment they are functioning in, and a high staff turnover often precludes this. Team goals may not be achieved if too few people are included for reasons of time. An effective team involved in a project will work through all the difficulties in some depth. Davies (1991) describes an instance of this when a contract was awarded to the cheapest bid. The contract overran as time had not been taken within the team to work out the detail of the contract.

There does not appear to be any research on the issue of gender and the effect of predominantly female teams on their effectiveness. Most health care professionals are female and may therefore be less assertive and expected to fulfil certain team functions. Leadership and vision are usually left to the leader – often the doctor and often male.

Knowledge and training in group dynamics is often part of the core curriculum for health professionals so that they start their professional life with knowledge of the concept and functioning of teams. This is not the case in industry and Anderson (1993) gives many reasons why training is essential

Practice point
Keep to:
- 3–10 team members
- split large teams, possibly with a common co-ordinator
- provide adequate time
- provide appropriate training
- develop clear professional roles

for teams in industry. Training opportunities exist for the development of interpersonal skills but there is perhaps insufficient training focusing on the teams themselves.

TEAM ROLES

It would seem inevitable for problems to arise between the professional groups if there is a blurring of roles, no clear idea of who does what and a lack of co-ordination. The professions therefore have:

- a poor idea of the role of the other
- insecurity leading to territoriality
- no means of conflict resolution
- incidental leadership.

Nurses, for example, often see themselves as core or essential to the patient care but separate from the team. In my recent experience of establishing ward-based teams for medical and elderly services, the steering group agreed, after some initial resistance from the consultants, that the ward sisters/charge nurses could be the team leaders rather than the consultants. The nurse managers, however, did not wish to assume the role and expressed concern that they had insufficient leadership skills. The nurses saw themselves as a team and the professions allied to medicine as the multidisciplinary team. The professions allied to medicine tend to be protective of their roles, although the need for such highly skilled people to undertake relatively routine tasks has been questioned by Gourlay (1991), the professions being the focus of service development rather than the patient.

Doctors still have a primary interest in diagnosis, and pressure to empty beds in acute hospitals re-enforces their commitment to medical stability rather than a more holistic model of physical and mental well-being with the emphasis on independence at home.

In all areas of health care the professions have little opportunity to learn the part each is expecting to play. This is partly because their education is essentially completed in different institutes; although there are now some faculties of health sciences, these do not include all disciplines. Assumptions are therefore made about the role of each team member, with subsequent stereotyping, which in turn leads to inflexibility. With many different professional groups involved with one patient, too many people can be involved in providing very small parts of the total package. Conversely, all the skills are over utilized when everyone assesses and treats the same problem area.

Ovretveit (1993) identifies five main problems occurring in multiprofessional teams:

- no care co-ordination
- deskilling
- contested role overlap
- reduced role autonomy
- role overload.

No care co-ordination

There is no clear accountability for the delivery of care to ensure that the agreed package of care is delivered to the patient. This can be solved by appointing a key worker or care manager with responsibility for individual patients.

Deskilling

In this case the team members are taking over other roles of case management or supervision and have little time to exercise their own professional skills.

Contested role overlap

In this situation two or more team members do the same work, which results in either a duplication of the work, or its not being done at all, each person assuming the other has done it, since both are able to.

Deciding who does the work if anyone could do it equally well, one profession may question whether another has the skills and knowledge to do it.

Reduced role autonomy

Clinicians used to working independently find they have less autonomy in the team. Different levels of autonomy have to be recognized even though this cuts across the egalitarian status of the team.

Role overload

Team members are unclear about their priorities and are undertaking too much of the wrong kind of work. They can also be members of different teams with too many responsibilities.

SUCCESSFUL TEAMS

A new model from Thomas (1992) for teams in primary health care shows teams moving across a spectrum from worst to assumed best in five stages.

- **Isolation** The team has no goals, no communication, restricted professional roles for team members and professional autonomy.
- **Awareness** The team has the intention to communicate but a lack of planning, team members have expectations and assumptions of roles, thus reinforcing status differences and making them reactive rather than proactive.
- **Proximation** The team has an acceptance of multi-disciplinary teams and planned communication, but members still have loose accountability with little interaction of specific tasks, i.e. no multidisciplinary assessments or home visits and some role conflict. The doctor tends to be the team leader.
- **Co-ordination** The team not only has planned goals but was itself selected and planned. Communication is more formalized, allowing for the exchange of views and ideas.
- **Dovetailing** The team skills are not role-bound and the patient and carer are in the team. Open communication and interpersonal trust is evident, allowing for conflict resolution.

Although the last stage may appear perfect, there is always the danger of the team becoming complacent and too inward looking, therefore not remaining aware of developments in their field outside their immediate environment.

LEADERSHIP

In health care the professionals are generally well motivated to achieving their professional goals. The team leader is essential for fulfilling the team goals rather than the professional goals and making sure that the patient/client is the focus of these goals.

Any team needs a leader, and successful teams have an identified leader and achieve their objectives. Ovretveit

---

Team leaders
A team leader is essential:
- for team goals
- to creat a client focus

(1993) claims that more team problems arise because of inadequate leadership than for any other reason. He believes this is the case not because the leader is inadequate for the work, but because the role is not clear or right for the type of team.

He uses the three concepts of responsibility, accountability and authority to clarify the team leadership role. He also finds it strange when health professionals with an in-depth knowledge of team functioning expect teams to function without a leader. The leadership role has to be made explicit to avoid the following problems:

- professional managers overcontrolling their staff, making it difficult for the team to function
- under control of staff assuming the team leader is managing them
- fuzzy accountability between the line manager and the team leader
- staff unclear who makes the decisions
- staff setting their own agenda because of poor decision making
- team leader's authority to uphold team policy is unclear
- channels for complaints are unclear.

Ovretveit defines three types of team leader roles:

- the elected team chairman
- the appointed team co-ordinator
- the appointed team manager.

When these three roles are discussed in terms of responsibility, accountability and authority no problems exist. It is when the leader is neither elected nor appointed but assumed or self-selected that problems arise and neither the team members nor the leader are clear about the leadership role.

According to Adair (1987), a good leader is directive in a democratic way, recalls the group to the strengthening unity of a common purpose, and makes the parts whole. Adair's list of the characteristics of good leadership with their associated outcomes is shown in Table 10.3.

Adair identifies three circles of responsibility and believes these are the key to successful leadership. Achieving the task is not possible without a clear idea of what it is and how it will be achieved by members of the team. This model applies well to health care teams as developing the individual is given equal weight with building the team. Adair summarizes his

---

Leadership types
- elect a chairman
- appoint a co-ordinator
- appoint a team manager

Table 10.3 Characteristics of good leaders and associated outcomes

Characteristics	Outcomes
Enthuser	People are purposefully busy and everyone has a basis on which to judge priorities
Lives his/her values, such as integrity	Sense of excitement; people willing to take risks; people willing to take on high work loads; feelings of achievement
Leads by example	Consistency; followers know leader's values
Generates good leaders from his/her followers	Is trusted by his/her followers
Aware of his/her own behaviour and environment	People aspire to leader's example
Intellect to meet the needs of the job	
Aware of the needs of the group he/she is leading and the needs of individuals	The led start to lead; leader becomes less indispensable; people are delegated to, coached and supported
Exhibits trust in his/her followers	
Able to represent the organization to his/her people and his/her people to the organization	Followers feel they have some contribution to the aims and are committed to them

views thus: 'Team work is no accident, it is the by-product of good leadership.'

To get the best possible team, leaders appear to need specific interpersonal skills and the leader and the team need to be clear about the leadership role and its relationship with the team. So rather than have teams, we often seem to have groups of people supposedly all working together for the good of the patient.

TEAM DEVELOPMENT

Teams do not therefore just happen. They have to be built and developed. This can be achieved via communication, education and quality, including audit. Regular meetings should be held where all are encouraged to participate. An external facilitator might be useful to help the team decide on its values and goals. The leader may in fact require facilitation skills and the group as a whole may identify certain areas where their communication and interpersonal skills need developing. These may be in the areas of negotiation or assertion. Valuing every person's contribution is not always

---

Practice point
Building teams requires:
- communication
- education
- quality

easy and the developing of listening skills by all team members is seldom a wasted exercise. Open discussion about the role of the leader and the team members will clarify the decision making process. As the leader has to encourage open discussion, the team members have to respect the decisions made by the leader.

At an undergraduate level, with the development of faculties of health sciences, a greater understanding of the various roles will occur. Meanwhile, specific case presentations demonstrating the various methods of assessment and the knowledge and skills underlying the assessment process will emphasise the strengths of each profession. Journal clubs allow for a constant review of clinical advances and evaluations. Patient-focused case presentations allow each professional group to demonstrate its own specific contribution. There will be a whole host of routine tasks that have to be done and the development of care workers with national vocational qualifications (NVQs) should allow clinicians time to practise their clinical skills rather than routine jobs, e.g. giving out walking aids. Joint evaluation and research projects will also help develop interdisciplinary trust.

Operational standards for purchasers must now exist as part of the *Patient's Charter* (Department of Health, 1991). These standards will also play an important part in countering ageism and guaranteeing high quality care for elderly people. Agreeing together on standards for referral, assessment and discharge gives an understanding of the standard-setting process and the essential part that audit plays in monitoring these standards. Ownership is key to the value placed on standards by health professionals, and recognition by the team of team ownership will lay the foundation for setting clinical guidelines and protocols. Trust built up at this stage will make the next stage easier – the acceptance of outcome measures reflecting the impact the team's health care work had on the patient.

REFERENCES

Adair, J. (1987) *Effective Teambuilding*, Pan Books, London.

Anderson, L.K. (1993) Teams: Group Process, Success and Carriers. *Journal of Nursing Administration*, **23**(9), 15–18.

Belbin, M. (1981) *Management Teams: Why They Succeed or Fail*, Butterworth-Heinnemann, Oxford.

Belbin, M. (1993) *Team Roles at Work*, Butterworth-Heinemann, Oxford.

Cumberlege, J. (1986) *Neighbourhood Nursing: A Focus for Care*, HMSO, London.

Chaudhry-Lawton, R., Lawton, R., Murphy, K. and Terry, A. (1992) *Quality: Change Through Teamwork*, Century Business, London.

Davies, P. (1991) Perspectives: Teamwork is good for you? *TQM Magazine*, **3**(1), 5–6.

Department of Health (1987) *Promoting Better Health. The Government's Programme for Improving Primary Health Care*, Cm 249, HMSO, London.

Department of Health (1991) *The Patient's Charter*, HMSO, London.

Dyer, W.C. (1977) *Team Building: Issues and Alternatives*, Addison-Wesley, Reading, MA.

Gourlay, R. (1991) Reprofiling the labour force. *International Journal of Health Care*, **4**(1), 3–6.

Katzenbach, J.R. and Smith, D.K. (1993) The discipline of teams. *Harvard Business Review*, **71**(2), 111–20.

Magerison, P. and McCann, A. (1987) *The Team Management Index*, MCB Press, Buckingham.

Navarro, V. (1987) *Medicine Under Capitalism*, Croom Helm, London.

Ovretveit, J. (1993) *Co-ordinating Community Care: Multidisciplinary Teams and Care Management*, Open University Press, Milton Keynes, p. 9.

Pritchard, P. (1995) Learning to work effectively in teams, in *Interprofessional Issues in Community and Primary Health Care*, (eds P. Owens, J. Carrier and J. Horder), Macmillan Press, London.

Reason, P. (1991) Power and conduct in multidisciplinary collaboration. *Complimentary Medical Research*, **5**(3), 144–50.

Spencer, J. and Pruss, A. (1992) *Managing Your Team: How to Organise People for Maximum Results*, Piatkus, London.

Thomas, M. (1992) *Approaches to Multiprofessional Learning in Continuing Education*. PhD thesis, University of Dundee.

Tuckman, B.W. (1965) Developmental sequences in small groups. *Psychology Bulletin*, **63**, 385–92.

Tuckman, B.W. and Jensen, M.A. (1977) Stages of small group development revisited. *Group Organizations Studies*, **2**, 419–27.

Training for quality 11

David L. Sandler and
Martin Sandler

EDITORS' INTRODUCTION

Previous chapters in this section have described the views of the individual professional groups that make up the multidisciplinary team.

This chapter describes the training available to those disciplines in the UK and elsewhere, but recognizes that there are severe difficulties in defining objectives, setting standards and monitoring the outcomes of education so as to define good quality. The chapter goes on to suggest that proxy measures such as identifying areas of poor care, the outcomes of examinations and health care research may help in definition.

The chapter points out that, although there is increasing international recognition for individual disciplines to obtain specialized education, often driven by the 'demographic explosion', there is as yet little multidisciplinary training available; and without good quality multidisciplinary management, good quality care is not obtainable. If multidisciplinary education is introduced early in professional training, there is a marked improvement in attitude, with less stereotyping and a more positive view of care interventions for elderly people.

Key topics
- Introduction
- Medicine for older people
- Nursing education
- Social work
- Therapy services
- Other aspects of training

INTRODUCTION

Determining quality is difficult, especially where outcomes are unclear or difficult to measure. Geriatric medicine itself is a heterogeneous specialty with poorly defined boundaries. Consequently, education within the field of care of elderly

Practice point
Move from example-based experience to objective-based training

Quality Care for Elderly People. Edited by Peter P. Mayer, Edward J. Dickinson and Martin Sandler. Published in 1997 by Chapman & Hall, London. ISBN 0 412 61830 3

people has been somewhat nebulous, its quality variable and unmeasured. As training in the care of elderly people evolves from example-based experience to established objective-based training, this situation is improving dramatically.

We consider here some aspects of quality in geriatric education as it relates to the elderly care team and its component specialties; we draw on the experience of the health care systems in the UK and elsewhere.

In training and education quality is important, but it is there that consensus ends – defining, measuring and implementing quality as an abstract concept is much more difficult. One definition of quality in training might be to define it as training to 'standards agreed by trainers skilled in the process, in an environment suitable to the task' (Pietroni, 1993). It rapidly becomes clear why it is problematic to define quality in geriatric education. Standards vary among people, institutions and regions, as do training skills and the educational and working environments. Additionally, we cannot be content simply to set these standards – there is a need to monitor the standards objectively with regard to processes, structure and outcome if quality education is to result and subsequently to develop further.

High standard care for elderly people requires a multidisciplinary approach, intrinsic to which is investment in the training of specialist nurses, therapists and medical social workers. A range of standards and initiatives designed to improve quality of training and care within the setting of an elderly care department is required.

QUALITY IN MEDICINE FOR ELDERLY PEOPLE

Training in elderly medicine began in the UK with the development of geriatric medicine as a specialty some 50 years ago. Since then, active training programmes have existed in the UK in both service and academic departments, with the first Chair of Geriatric Medicine in the world being established in Glasgow in 1965.

Specific training in medicine for elderly people in North America and its recognition as a specialty lagged behind the UK, with only 15 medical schools in the USA teaching geriatric medicine or gerontology in 1976. This increased by the late 1980s to give a total of 102 schools that included gerontology or geriatric courses in their curriculum out of 126 schools.

Setting standards
- Multidisciplinary
- Different settings
- Adequate monitoring

Recognition of elderly medicine as a specialty on mainland Europe has also been slow in comparison with Britain, with few countries recognizing medicine for elderly people as a specific entity in the medical school teaching syllabus.

In Japan there are only 13 academic departments of geriatric medicine out of a total of 80 medical schools, the first independent department of geriatric medicine having been established in Tokyo in 1962.

Despite the relatively advanced state of current training arrangements in the UK, there are nevertheless some well documented shortcomings in the medical care of elderly people. These include the underdiagnosis of a number of medical disorders (Williamson, 1981), over- and inappropriate prescribing (Tulloch, 1981), poor management of disability and sensory impairment (Tulloch and Moore, 1979; Patrick, Peach and Gregg, 1982), lack of attention to proper instruction of patients with regard to physical aids (George et al., 1988) as well as inadequate attention paid to carer needs and stress (Hicks, 1988).

> **Shortcomings in care**
> - Underdiagnosis
> - Prescribing drugs and aids
> - Carer needs
> - Prevention

Similarly, the area of preventative medicine in elderly medicine is poorly taught. It is argued that this is because most undergraduate and postgraduate medical teaching is undertaken in a hospital setting and not in primary care. The link between education and medical care is at present enigmatic. It is, however, uncertain whether the diagnosis and management of other conditions or other age groups is handled any better.

These research findings may be regarded as rough outcome measures for medical education relating to elderly people. Such information stimulates questions about training and its quality, particularly about the methodology used for assessment of medical education, both at the undergraduate and postgraduate level.

In the UK, the General Medical Council is responsible for the monitoring of undergraduate curricula. It inspects changes in medical schools' syllabuses in an effort to maintain standards and uniformity between the different institutions. It is also responsible for ensuring the educational standards of doctors trained abroad who wish to practise in the UK.

All UK medical schools now have active departments of medicine for the elderly which contribute to the undergraduate curricula. Increasingly, departments of primary care medicine also provide a more balanced and appropriate education for current and recent undergraduates. Early

> **Practice point**
> Early exposure of medical students decreases stereotyping

exposure of medical students to elderly patients has been shown to reinforce positive attitudes to ageing and tends to decrease stereotyping (Shahidi and Devlen, 1993), which is detrimental to the care of elderly people.

Postgraduate training for non-career grade doctors has been considered to be of particular importance given that this group of trainees includes those going on to other specialties and those entering primary care. A recent joint report of the Royal College of Physicians (1994) and the British Geriatric Society suggested minimum standards of training for those non-specialists looking after elderly people with medical illnesses. As part of training in internal (general) medicine, the report recommends that a period of six months should be spent in geriatric medicine with experience of all the various component parts of the service. Likewise, in training as a specialist geriatrician, a significant period of time should be spent in general medicine. The Training Committee of the British Geriatric Society has recommended a core curriculum of learning objectives for the training of such individuals. The principles of good geriatric medical care are additionally cascading down to doctors in training from general physicians who have been trained in medicine for the elderly but who are employed as general physicians with special responsibility for the elderly.

Additionally, it has been suggested that individuals who take on particular responsibilities in a primary care setting (e.g. medical supervision of nursing homes) should demonstrate particular skills in medicine for the elderly. The Diploma in Geriatric Medicine has been suggested as an appropriate criterion.

Postgraduate training of the senior and career registrars has been the responsibility of the Joint Committee for Higher Medical Training with input from the British Geriatric Society and the Royal College of Physicians of London (Swift and James, 1991). The basic components of training in medicine for the elderly in the UK include acute geriatric care, continuing care, rehabilitation (including orthogeriatric rehabilitation), day hospital work, domiciliary assessment and experience of psychiatry for elderly people. In addition, an important part of training has been the participation in research, teaching and the acquisition of managerial skills. In recent surveys, senior registrars in the UK (Sandler, Castledon and Ritch, 1991) have expressed some concerns about the quality of their training in terms of research in geriatric medicine, psychiatry of the elderly and health

Basic training
- Acute care
- Continuing care
- Rehabilitation
- Day hospitals
- Domiciliary assessment

service management. These findings were mirrored by a further survey of newly appointed consultants (Sandler, 1992) that enquired about the relevance and adequacy of their training experience in geriatric medicine.

The content of career grade education in geriatric medicine has also recently been looked at by the British Geriatric Society, which identified the relevant components of training and made recommendations. Many of the career grade rotational posts have subsequently been enhanced, but attempts to determine the quality of education still remain elusive. At present, monitoring depends on subjective achievement of objectives. However, this may at least be regarded as a platform upon which to build and may avoid the concept of exit examinations.

Training for career grade doctors in psychiatry has been developing along similar lines. The advent of the requirement for continuing medical education (CME) as directed by the Royal College of Physicians in the UK may also have a beneficial impact on the continuing education of career doctors, including consultants. It is too early to assess how beneficial CME might prove.

There are other attempts at standardizing and improving educational quality which, although not specific to geriatric medicine, may be beneficial. The King's Fund Organizational Audit is a national approach to improving the organization and delivery of health care through the setting and monitoring of standards. At present, some 180 'units' are involved in this audit both in the private and NHS sectors. The educational standards audited by the King's Fund include staff development and educational arrangements. The audit is designed to facilitate professional progression and the way in which it relates to service needs in conjunction with the overall needs of the organization. The audit consists of core objectives, but also specific clinically-based criteria. It encourages the setting of standards including monitoring of training, supervision of junior doctors, provision of relevant educational material and monitoring of CME among career grade doctors.

In the USA, various interested bodies including the American Geriatric Society, the Institute of Medicine and the Executive Council of the Association of American Medical Colleges are strong proponents of the incorporation of gerontology and geriatric medicine into the medical school curriculum. However, they are still not mandatory subjects in the undergraduate teaching programme of a significant proportion of medical schools in the USA, despite evidence to suggest

Areas that are badly taught
• Psychiatry
• Research
• Management

Organizational audit
• Standards
• Core objectives
• Clinical criteria
• Monitoring of training

that education, and therefore quality care, can only come with significant exposure to the constituent parts of geriatric care.

Different initiatives have evolved in North America with regard to training in geriatric medicine. Primarily as a response to the 'demographic explosion' expected in the USA, the Geriatric Research, Education and Clinical Centers (GRECCs) were created (Goodwin and Morley, 1994). The idea behind their inception was that improved care of elderly people would follow if clinical care, research and education were situated in a common locus. By 1994, some 16 centres had been established in close association with established medical schools, and 'ongoing assessment programmes' had been instituted by the Veterans' Affairs Central Office by way of monitoring their effectiveness in research and education.

The GRECCs have been responsible for a large proportion of the research into elderly people in the USA, but they also function as centres of excellence, training both undergraduate and postgraduate students in geriatric care. They have also been responsible for the promotion of research into health service management and have promoted the concept of quality in the care of elderly people in the USA.

Postgraduate education in the USA and its quality is controlled by the Accreditation Council for Graduate Medical Education which is responsible for the Geriatric Fellowship Programs. Certification requirements have resulted in increasing numbers of geriatricians applying for continuing medical education programmes. These are a function of the Bureau of Health Professions via its Geriatric Education Centers programme.

> **GRECCS**
> Establishing clinical care, research and education in one locus

QUALITY AND NURSING EDUCATION

In the UK, nursing education has, and is still, undergoing tremendous changes in both pre- and postregistration training. The United Kingdom Central Council (UKCC) considers quality in education to be of great importance (UKCC, 1986, 1989) and nursing educationalists are increasingly vigorous in the quest to enhance and develop training appropriate to the changing demands of nursing.

Similarly, integrating quality gerontological nursing education into the baccalaureate curriculum of American schools of nursing (Nelson, 1992) has become an urgent necessity

in view of the expected demographic changes in the elderly
population in the USA. Such integration has been recommended for a number of years, though it has been slow to
occur, partly because of a reluctance to make changes to the
curriculum (Joel, 1987; ANA, 1982). It was feared that such
alterations might make individual nurse training programmes
less attractive, and that recruitment might suffer.

In a 1984 study (Edel, 1986), only 4.41% of nursing faculties
out of 197 institutions in the USA had undertaken any
coursework in geriatrics or gerontology. There are increasing
efforts, however, to include gerontological nursing and clinical experience in undergraduate programmes, in addition to
increasing the number of 'elderly friendly' teachers and lecturers (ANA, 1986; Hogstel, 1988; Malliarakis and Heine,
1990).

> **Core nurse training**
> - Successful ageing
> - Health promotion
> - Disease processes

There are a number of programmes in the USA whose
primary aim is to improve the quality of gerontological nursing education. For example, the Faculty Preparation for
Teaching Gerontological Nursing project, sponsored by the
Southern Regional Education Board, was specifically designed for this purpose. Its aim is to acquaint nursing college
lecturers with current gerontological practice and research
and their future implications via a series of workshops. The
core curriculum plan incorporates elements relating to successful ageing as well as health promotion for elderly people.
It also includes topics relating to the differing pathological
processes and presentation of disease in elderly people.

In the UK, nursing the elderly may have been viewed nega-
tively, and the paucity of postregistration courses available
in gerontology, compared with those in 'high tech' nursing,
bears sad testament to the perception of nursing elderly
people as a 'Cinderella' specialty (Dyer, 1993). In an attempt
to increase the quality of gerontological education in nursing,
a number of steps have been taken, and there has been an
increased emphasis on standards in nursing education *per se*,
which probably dates back to 1984 and Maxwell's paper
(Maxwell, 1984) on quality assessment in health.

Maxwell's dimensions of quality are: access, relevance,
effectiveness, equity, social acceptability and efficiency and
economy. As a model of quality, it can be used to test education in a logical and systematic fashion. It is increasingly used
to assess educational processes as well as strategies in health
care. Developing in a fashion that is complementary to the
improvements in educational standards and quality has been
an increase in the number of postregistration courses in

gerontology-related subjects (though not at the same rate as non-gerontological courses!). They are presently based in a variety of educational institutions in the UK and go to diploma, masters level or beyond. Additionally, a number of nursing colleges are responding to the need to integrate with higher education and improve their educational standards by upgrading the academic content of their gerontology course. This might, of course, be in response to the English Nursing Board's higher award initiative, which now assesses and allocates credits to individual courses.

One novel initiative to improve the quality of nursing education in the care of elderly people, has been the Royal College of Nursing (RCN) update distance learning project. As a way of keeping nurses up to date, and mindful of postregistration needs in education and practice, the RCN has utilized its own journal (*Nursing Standard*) and nationally transmitted television programmes to develop an easily accessible distance learning medium that it is hoped will result in an improvement in the quality of geriatric education among the RCN's members.

Another example of such an initiative is in Australia, where nurses involved in the care of elderly people developed a special group (Nay-Brock, 1988) to promote the specialty of nurses in geriatric care. Since the 1980s this group has expanded to include state enrolled nurses and nursing assistants, and subsequently to involve those working in nursing homes. Through educational programmes, regular meetings and the exchange of ideas and information, educational standards have improved, as has the quality of geriatric nursing care.

The establishment in the UK of National Vocational Qualifications (NVQs) has resulted in a common training base as well as a framework for joint training throughout both statutory and non-statutory organizations. Certain voluntary organizations, e.g. Age Concern, Crossroads, have developed strong training arrangements not only for themselves but also for informal carers.

Quality examples
- RCN distance learning project
- Australian special group development

British Association of Social Workers
Special skills in:
- relationships
- bereavement
- complex multidisciplinary problems

QUALITY, CARE OF ELDERLY PEOPLE AND MEDICAL SOCIAL WORK

Social workers are an integral part of the multidisciplinary team and play an important role in the delivery of care to elderly people in hospital and in the community. Before the advent of social service departments in the UK, most of the work in this field was done by largely unqualified welfare officers (Tinker, 1992). In contrast, most social workers for children were specifically trained and worked with direct support from paediatric departments. Changes towards a more generic approach to training in social work were mooted in 1959 (MoH/DoH, 1959) and 1968 (DoES, 1968).

By 1986, there was a return to client group specialization, with elderly people being disadvantaged in a variety of ways (Rowlings, 1981). The Younghusband Committee (1959) had previously clarified the role of the geriatric social worker as a professional providing a means for assessing problems and instituting appropriate practical assistance if possible. In 1977, the British Association of Social Workers laid down guidelines for working with and providing support to elderly clients (BASW, 1977). They suggest that there is a need for expertise in elderly social work in the same way as for other age groups, and that proper training is essential for the delivery of a quality service. The guidelines place particular emphasis on the need to acquire special skills for helping with relationships and bereavement in elderly people, as well as for coping with the complex problems arising from the interplay of medical, social and psychological factors in elderly people.

Recent policy developments have resulted in an increasing training requirement for social workers in the role of care manager. This is as a consequence of the NHS and Community Care Act, 1990, and also due to an increase in the demands of working with a growing number of dementia sufferers and carers requiring support, and negotiating with other agencies and advocating for patients' rights. In what is becoming a recurrent theme, only proper attention to training can develop social workers with the appropriate skills to deliver quality input to their clients and thus provide excellent care to elderly people.

QUALITY AND THERAPISTS

The need for therapists who have relevant training and experience of working with elderly people is increasing with the change in age structure of most developed countries. Training may be at diploma or degree level, and postgraduate degrees are available in a number of institutions. In previous years, therapists working with elderly people may have seen

Holistic educational needs
- Social
- Medical
- Psychological
- Early exposure

little need for a specific gerontological content to their education, but today's professionals would tend to disagree (Peterson and Wendt, 1990).

In the USA, the 1981 White House Conference on Ageing emphasized that quality care for elderly people requires well educated health professionals, and that people delivering these services require specific gerontological training. In North America, specific areas of educational need have been identified (Cryns and Wilderdom, 1989) in professionals working with elderly people. These include the social aspects of their care as well as the specific medical and psychological problems associated with growing older. A survey of entry level educational programmes for therapists in the USA in 1990 found that 89% of courses had a specific gerontology component within the course itself. Other studies have found that early exposure of therapy students to elderly patients in sufficient numbers does in fact positively affect the students' attitudes to elderly people, the implications of which are clear.

OTHER RELEVANT ASPECTS OF QUALITY IN EDUCATION

Practice point
High quality care of elderly people requires high quality education of the multidisciplinary team

Individual disciplines have been singled out and aspects of their training dissected. One key message for practitioners in the care of elderly people is that these are components of the greater multidisciplinary team. No single discipline is sufficient in itself to deliver high quality care. There is, however, no formalized training on how best to develop or lead these multidisciplinary teams, and little education, other than experience, on how to approach the various situations that arise within the individual teams.

As more teamwork is required in both institutional and community care, there will be a greater need for training in leadership and communication skills, as well as in team building. Training in aspects of management is noted to be lacking in surveys of senior registrars and newly appointed consultants. Many of the rotational training schemes currently encourage attendance at management courses to help reduce that shortfall. More structured management training for doctors, and probably other groups of clinical staff, in the UK will be necessary as clinicians' involvement in management increases. Indeed, it may not be long before Medical Management emerges as a subspecialty in its own right.

It is worth briefly reversing the elements of the subject of this chapter to address 'education in quality'. Little formal training is given in assessment of the quality of care at present. The inception of medical audit was greeted with great enthusiasm, and significant resources were expended on developing projects to improve care. But at a time when there is no completely reliable and generally accepted medical language, and no means of coding severity, there has been little tangible advance in the quality of care. This might partly be due to a lack of training in audit principles and techniques. Training in quality assessment and development will need to become an integral part of the undergraduate and postgraduate curricula in the very near future.

CONCLUSION

Quality of education in the care of elderly people is hard to define. It remains virtually impossible to measure quality in elderly medical education in a direct or indirect fashion. Therefore quality in elderly medical education remains difficult to monitor, and proxy methods of estimating the outcome of such education, e.g. examinations, attendance records, health care research, remain in use. Some promising initiatives are being developed, but there is a need for initiatives and progress in other areas. It is clear that education remains the cornerstone of quality progression in the care of elderly people.

REFERENCES

American Nursing Association (1982) *A Challenge for Change: the role of gerontological nursing*, AMA, Division on Gerontological Nursing Practice, Kansas City.

American Nursing Association (1986) *Gerontological Nursing Curriculum: survey analysis and recommendations*, AMA, Kansas City.

British Association of Social Workers (1977) Statement. *Social Work Today*, 12 April, 13.

Committee on Strengthening the Geriatric Content of Medical Training (1994) Strengthening training in geriatrics for physicians. *Journal of the American Geriatric Society*, **42**, 559–65.

Cryns, A.G. and Wilderdom, C.P.M. (1989) Continuing education needs in geriatrics/gerontology: specifying occupational and organizational attributes of service professionals. *Educational Gerontology*, **15**, 81–101.

Department of Education and Science (1968) *The Seebholm Report: Report of the committee on local authority and allied personal social services*, HMSO, London.

Dyer, S. (1993) Gerontology: the sexy end of education. *Elderly Care*, **5**(3), 10–11.

Edel, M.K. (1986) Recognise gerontological content. *Journal of Gerontological Nursing*, **12**(10), 28–32.

George, J., Binns, V.E., Clayden, A.D. and Mulley, G.P. (1988) Aids and adaptations for the elderly at home: underprovided. *British Medical Journal*, **296**, 1365–6.

Goodwin, H. and Morley, J. (1994) Geriatric research, education and clinical centers: their impact in the development of American geriatics. *Journal of the American Geriatric Society*, **42**, 1012–19.

Hicks, C. (1988) *Who Cares: Looking After Old People at Home*, Virgo Press, Reading.

Hogstel, M. (1988) Gerontological nursing in the baccalaureate curriculum. *Nurse Educator*, **13**(3), 14–18.

Joel, L.A. (1987) *The geriatric imperative: entry level and graduate nursing education in models for long term care*, National League for Nursing Publication No 20-2188, 7–13.

Malliarakis, D.R. and Heine, C. (1990) Is gerontological nursing included in baccalaureate nursing programs? *Journal of Gerontological Nursing*, **16**(6), 4–7.

Maxwell, R.J. (1984) Quality assessment in health. *British Medical Journal*, **288**, 1740–2.

Nay-Brock, R. (1988) Future trends in the care of the elderly; aged care – the elements of a chapter. *The Australian Nurses' Journal*, **17**(9), 12–14, 34.

Nelson, M.K. (1992) Geriatric nursing in the baccalaureate curriculum. *Journal of Gerontological Nursing*, **18**(7), 26–30.

Patrick, D.L., Peach, H. and Gregg, I. (1982) Disablement and care: a comparison of patient views and GP knowledge. *Journal of the Royal College of General Practitioners*, **32**, 429–34.

Peterson, D. and Wendt, P. (1990) Employment in the fields of ageing: a survey of professionals in four fields. *The Gerontologist*, **30**(5), 479–84.

Pietroni, M. (1993) Quality in medical education and training. *British Journal of Hospital Medicine*, **49**(4), 237–46.

Rowlings, C. (1981) *Social Work with Elderly People*, Allen & Unwin, London.

Royal College of Physicians/British Geriatric Society (1994) *Ensuring Equity and Quality of Care of Elderly People: The Interface Between Geriatric and General Medicine*, RCP, London.

Sandler, M. (1992) Survey of recently appointed consultants in geriatric medicine. *Journal of the Royal College of Physicians of London*, **26**(1), 44–6.

Sandler, M., Castledon, B. and Ritch, A. (1991) Senior registrar training in geriatric medicine 1977–1990. *Journal of the Royal College of Physicians of London*, **25**(4), 304–5.

Shahidi, S. and Devlen, J. (1993) Medical students' attitudes to and knowledge of the aged. *Medical Education*, **27**, 286–8.

Swift, C.G. and James, O.F.W. (1991) *Training and manpower in geriatric medicine*. The British Geriatric Society Training Committee, London.

Tinker, A. (1992) A critical narrative of the main developments in social services for elderly people, in *Elderly People in Modern Society* (ed. A. Tinker), Longman, Harlow.

Tulloch, A.J. (1981) Repeat prescribing for elderly patients. *British Medical Journal*, **282**, 1672–5.

Tulloch, A.J. and Moore, V. (1979) A randomised controlled trial of geriatric screening in general practice. *Journal of the Royal College of General Practitioners*, **29**, 355–9.

Williamson, J. (1981) The Preventative Approach, in *The Provision of Care for the Elderly* (eds J. Kinnaird, J.H.F. Brotherstone and J. Williamson), Churchill Livingstone, Edinburgh.

UKCC (1986) Project 2000, A New Preparation for Practice, United Kingdom Central Council, London.

UKCC (1989) Information on Post-registration Education and Practice Project, United Kingdom Central Council, London.

Younghusband Committee (1959) *The Younghusband Report. Report of the working party on social workers in local authority health and welfare services*. Ministry of Health and Department of Health for Scotland, HMSO, London.

Part Four
Organizations

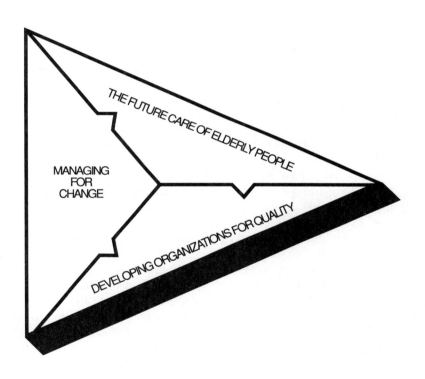

THE FUTURE CARE OF ELDERLY PEOPLE

MANAGING
FOR
CHANGE

DEVELOPING ORGANIZATIONS FOR QUALITY

EDITORS' INTRODUCTION TO PART FOUR

To achieve high quality care, people in their teams need the support of their organizations. Yet, as we saw in Part One, organizations face a constantly changing environment. In addition, Part Two showed us that organizations need to work with each other across sectors of care with differing perspectives, roles and responsibilities. Faced with these twin challenges, how can care organizations ensure that they are healthy and support their staff in delivering high quality care? And what philosophy should be pursued?

To answer this question, this part brings in the role of management and philosophy in achieving successful care. This is done by looking in turn at:

- how organizations can change
- how organizations can develop quality
- how organizations can respond and plan for the future.

An important underlying theme in this part of the book is that of the costs of care. If organizations do not change, they may become bureaucratic, dysfunctional and inefficient, squandering money unnecessarily. Almost all experience suggests that striving for high quality will actually reduce the costs of care. Similarly, resources will be used most wisely by working to a common philosophy. For example, it might be tempting for health providers to discontinue rehabilitation as, from their perspective, it is costly and unnecessary. It might also be tempting to limit the hospital care of elderly people because it is costly and complex. However, these approaches would be disastrous for society as a whole: they would lead to a rapid escalation in the costs of long-term care to an unsustainable level, because of the increased care needs for untreated and unrehabilitated elderly people.

Thus, in considering costs, wide and longer term perspectives are needed – although this is not an approach encouraged by present systems of organization and funding. The need for this approach is underlined by arguments about the costs of quality. Poor quality results in the costs of rework and failure. Ironically, these costs may not be felt ('as that's the way we do things around here') or they may be felt by others (for example, the human costs of pain or suffering). In health care, rework would best be seen in duplication of paperwork, assessments and records; failure would correspond to missed opportunities for health gain, complications and complaints. Tackling quality may demand changes and investment (of various resources – money, time, equipment) which might seem counter-intuitive at the outset, especially to practitioners. A commonly heard response is: 'I haven't got time for quality – I'm busy enough with my clients'. However, in time the benefits are in reduced costs of poor quality and lower costs of routine work.

Chapter 12 gives practical advice on achieving successful development of services with special emphasis on culture and people. Chapter 13 argues that centring attention on quality is a way of navigating the stormy waters of change using a limited number of realistic principles. Chapter 14 focuses on how services might respond constructively to future demographic challenges, concentrating on the need to spotlight the interface into long-term care from philosophical, mathematical and practical viewpoints.

By the end of this part, the reader will have an understanding of how organizations work and how they can contribute to the quality of care.

Managing for change 12

Peter S. Stansbie

EDITORS' INTRODUCTION

The following chapter – written by a President of the Institute of Health Service Management and a former Chief Executive of a West Midlands Health Authority and now Chief Executive of a large Health Authority in Wales – clearly recognizes that managing change is not easy. It acknowledges that the pace of change has increased dramatically over the past 10 years and that change cannot occur without health service staff being party to, accepting and leading that change.

This first chapter in this part of the book describes that change, the process of managing it, changing the culture and methods for bringing people into the process. The main message is perhaps embodied in the prayer on the author's office wall about the ability to accept the limitation imposed by time, resources and people but to provide the information, education and understanding that enables people to achieve, change objectives and enhance good quality care at all levels of the organization.

Key topics
- Continous change
- The process of managing change
- Changing the culture
- People

CONTINUOUS CHANGE

The past 10 years have seen continuous change in the National Health Service (NHS) at what often feels like a growing pace. We have to accept that change is not going to stop, is probably going to quicken in pace, and has to be managed. Unmanaged change is undirected and confused. Unless we do manage for change we will find we are less able to achieve the results we want and less able to provide excellent care.

Managing for change is about three things: people, people and people. If we had a production line that worked with

Quality Care for Elderly People. Edited by Peter P. Mayer, Edward J. Dickinson and Martin Sandler. Published in 1997 by Chapman & Hall, London. ISBN 0 412 61830 3

robots, managing for change would be easy. But in the NHS, and in caring for elderly people, that will never be the case. People do not like change, people resist change and people worry about change. But those same people deliver the services that we want to improve and, of course, deliver the changes. If we are to manage for change, and change which will continue, we have to recognize all the time that the process we are involved in centres on people.

This chapter looks at why we need to manage for change, the sort of change that is occurring now and may occur in the future, and the structure, processes and culture within which we have to work. It then sets out some practical suggestions on how we might manage for change, and particularly manage people for change.

CHANGE NOW

Causing change
- Legislation
- Society
- Technology
- Skills

For the past 10 years, change has affected the NHS and the care of elderly people with increasing pace. This change has come through legislation, societal change and technological and skills changes. Major initiatives have included community care, a huge increase in the number of private nursing homes and residential care establishments, a move towards improved packages of care in the home, and changes to the structure and culture of the NHS.

In addition, there has been a managerial revolution in the NHS, which has seen the implementation of general management, a move away from consensus management (although I hope this will be re-invented), and greater awareness of the quality and costs of patient care than we have seen before.

As if that was not enough, we are finding an increased general interest in health and health care. This follows society's move towards consumerism and a much greater awareness of health and health care in the general population. We are not immune from such changes, and, indeed, should not be immune from them. There is now not one national newspaper, either broadsheet or tabloid, that does not have a regular health column in its pages every week.

Box 12.1 lists the main changes of the past 12 years, although you may want to add your own changes to this list.

All of these factors increase the pressure for change and the need to manage it. Given this, it is not surprising that management has developed its own processes and systems to

---

Box 12.1   Main NHS changes 1984–1996

- General management
- Purchaser–provider split
- NHS trusts
- Reduction in hospital beds
- Growth in nursing homes
- Care in the community
- Hospital at home
- Health commissions
- Reduction in the number of hours worked by junior hospital doctors
- Reskilling
- Consumerism
- Increased cost pressures
- New combined HAs
- Primary care-led NHS
- PM suggests joint health/social services mental health authorities

---

capture the management of change. Current 'systems' that capture this mood and are always useful to quote when trying to impress people about change include:

- process re-engineering
- total quality management (TQM)
- continuous quality improvement (CQI)
- patient-centred care.

In fact all of these systems simply put a framework around the process of managing change in a way that concentrates on the consumer and allows substantial cultural change within the organization.

Practice point
Systems provide a framework for cultural change

CHANGE IN THE FUTURE

We are bound to see more of the same. Changes in technology, changes in skills and knowledge, increased consumer awareness and continuing financial pressures mean that ongoing change will continue. While we may have seen the end of the major legislative changes in health care, we will continue to see internal and external changes for the foreseeable future.

Challenges
- Few hospital beds
- Improved care at home

Practice point
Leadership and effective teams are crucial

Practice point
Involve people affected in setting clear objectives with measurable outcomes

The current situation looks 'challenging' for all of us. We will see pressure for fewer hospital beds, matched by pressure for improved care in the home and primary care settings. The fragile line between health and social care also looks increasingly challenged. So we could well see changes in structures as well as changes in working patterns within the current structures.

I am also confident that in the future we will see an increase in nurse practitioners, and perhaps other health care professionals, challenging the medical profession for its historical lead in delivering health care.

However, whatever changes mean, the delivery of excellent care will continue to demand strong and effective teams of people. Health care is complex and its delivery is often more so. While individuals with different skills are vital to the process, they are more powerful when they work together in teams. Leadership of those teams is crucially important, but where that leadership comes from is less important.

Management will increasingly become leadership, with different people from different backgrounds taking on this role in a variety of different settings. It is these leaders of the future who will have to manage all the change that will occur, and manage the people who deliver care to the people who receive it, in such a way that change is not undirected, painful and ineffective.

THE PROCESS OF MANAGING CHANGE

So change will happen and change is about people. How then do we want to manage it?

The aim of managing change is to make it effective, smooth and directed towards the goals we are trying to achieve. A simple process for managing change is shown in Box 12.2. Now this process looks simple. And it is! At least it would be if we were not dealing with people.

Firstly, people do not like being challenged on what they are trying to achieve. People like to involve themselves in processes and doing things. Stopping and asking ourselves what we are trying to achieve and setting clear objectives is both difficult and time consuming, but of course if we do not do it, we cannot manage the process of change. In particular we must be clear about the outcomes we wish to achieve and when we want to achieve them; and they must be measurable. Too often people set loose goals, move towards them

---

Box 12.2   A process for managing change

1. Ask – what do we want to achieve?
2. Write down clear objectives:
   • **what** do we want?
   • **when** do we want it?
   • **how** will we know we have got there?
3. Thaw the organization.
4. Consider the 'externals'.
5. Refreeze it in new shape.
6. Try it.
7. Review outcomes and processes.
8. Be prepared to change again.

---

and then wonder why nothing happens. So we need to sit down with all the people concerned and work through with them what we are trying to achieve, when we are trying to achieve it and how we will know we have succeeded.

At this point it is important to stress that the people doing the job are the best people to know what needs to change and how best to change it. It is no good for managers and supervisors to just sit down with this process, we must involve all our staff in finding ways of doing it. Again, this sounds simple, but is in fact very difficult. People are very conscious of status and position, and some people are much better at expressing themselves than others. But investing time in this process will make all the difference at the end of the day.

One way of carrying out this process is by using quality circles. This is a system developed in the USA and Japan for involving workers in quality improvement. North Warwickshire NHS Trust has successfully used this approach in a wide variety of settings. Basically, quality circles involve a facilitated group of people from a specific area, e.g. a ward. They work together to identify problems and then tackle a particular problem and make a presentation to management with solutions. Practical results of such a process can be quite startling. Across North Warwickshire NHS Trust there have been major improvements in ward areas and service areas, and significant improvements in service.

The scheme has been operating in the trust since 1984 and continues today. Areas that have been reviewed include: two wards for elderly people in a small hospital, and links

Quality circles
• Identify problem
• Tackle it
• Present solutions to management
• Involve staff
• Save money
• Improve quality

between the hospital and community services, including the provision of a 'tea and tub' service, which brings patients into the hospital for the day and gives them tea and a bath.

A facilitator works to develop the programme and works with the circles themselves, ensuring that the people doing the job are indentifying the problems and solving them. One of the important factors about the use of quality circles is that as well as improving quality, they can also save money. Although this is not their main purpose, they do prove that improvements in quality can be achieved at low cost or indeed with a saving.

Other areas of Warwickshire have also used quality circles including George Eliot Hospital NHS Trust, which successfully used the process to improve its day services for elderly people.

The next part of this process is starting to 'thaw' the organization. People working together get very set in the patterns in which they operate. If we are to make effective change we have to start loosening the processes and structures that tie us to the existing patterns. This is often a painful process. We are challenging people's status and position in the organization and asking them to challenge it too. Not surprisingly, people cling to what they know and what they think they are good at. We have to enable people to recognize that what they are doing and the way they are doing it is not always perfect, and that it can be challenged by them and by others. If we can engage people in a culture that allows change and changes in position to take place without a loss of status, we will have achieved much.

In involving people in change and enabling us to 'thaw' the organization, it is necessary to take time out from the normal day-to-day processes. Given that the work in health care just goes on and cannot be stopped like a production line, doing this can be quite difficult. However, we must find the time to bring people together to talk, to discuss, to learn, and to set an agreed agenda. We cannot do this without taking limited but protected time away from the day-to-day workload. It only needs to be half an hour, but it needs to be focused and produce ideas for measurable change so that we can monitor our own performance.

Again, I cannot stress too much the need to bring the people actually doing the job together in these circumstances. They will need to be led in the process by someone, not necessarily their natural manager, who can facilitate the process in a non-threatening way and ensure that progress is monitored by the people themselves whenever they meet.

Practice point
Enable people to challenge themselves

Bringing people together
- Facilitator
- Time out
- Focused
- Self-monitored

Setting small tasks and making small changes often does more to 'thaw' an organization than trying to tackle major change all in one go. Nothing succeeds like success, and this enables people, particularly those who may be anxious or opposed to change, to see some benefit and also to start generating their own ideas.

At this stage it is also important to consider the external pressures being faced by the organization. Some of these pressures can be changed or modified, but many others cannot. There is no point in trying to change external pressure because it is something over which you have no control or power. You need to understand such pressures and accept them as a reality. Too often, time and effort is diverted away from positive change by trying to change what cannot be altered, and of course, this failure frustrates your own change.

The most common external problem, perceived and real, is a lack of resources. Now, every person leading change has a responsibility to obtain the maximum resource possible for his or her part of the organization. If, however, resources cannot be increased, then you have to recognize that fact and work with what you have got. Trying to gain more resource when it is just not available is frustrating and debilitating. So look at the available resource and how it could be better used.

Recognizing that external changes are often beyond your own power and influence is an important part of the change process and can lead to a recognition that internal change is not only necessary but desirable. It can often help with changes to existing structures when people recognize that they are more in control of their own destiny than that of the outside world.

Recognizing external pressures and influences often forces you to look more closely at what is happening and available within your own setting. It can often lead to a recognition that you can do more for yourselves, and therefore to an ability and wish to change that can lead to a startling transformation.

We can now look at what is needed to achieve our aims and involve staff in shaping the new structure needed to achieve them. Only after this can we then 'freeze' the organization back into a new shape in which it can start to achieve its new goals. We do have to put a new structure around what we are trying to do as people find it difficult to cope without structure and do like to know what they are doing and to whom they are reporting.

- Aim to succeed
- Make small changes often

External pressures
- Alter the alterable
- Do not strive after the impossible

Practice point
- New shapes require new structures
- Set a date for the changes if possible

So, having worked through what we are trying to achieve, established clear objectives, worked through with people how we can change (five minutes on paper and five months in doing it!) we then have to try our new situation. It is quite often useful when doing this to set a date for the changes to be implemented. We cannot always do this, but if we can it does help with people's feeling of security and actually gives quite a 'buzz' if it is handled well.

We now need to allow some time for the new structures and systems to 'bed in' and for people to learn to work with them. There is often a tendency to pull the new flower up and look at its roots before it has had time to grow. If this happens, of course, the flower could easily die. So allow some time before the next stage, which is review.

Review is necessary to judge whether the changes have been successful. People need time to settle into what they are doing and for the changes to work, but after a while, do review the changes, and review them together. Check the outcomes and the processes and then the most difficult thing of all: **be prepared to change again**.

It is all too easy, having worked through a difficult and time-consuming process of change, to stick with that change at all costs and not make small, simple additional changes that will make all the difference. Again, if you involve the people doing the job, they will often do some of this for themselves, but if you do not involve them they will carry on doing what they have been asked to do and they will know very well it is wrong.

One of the strongest measures of leadership is being prepared to accept that you were wrong and that you need to change. Generally, the culture in the NHS does not find accepting mistakes easy. Yet the only people who do not make mistakes are people who are not doing anything. It is crucial that we start to accept the mistakes that we and others make, and that we should not be torn limb from limb as a result of them, if we are to make the change process work.

If people are genuinely trying to do something new and different, and they make a mistake, that is the very point at which you have to learn together what has happened and not criticize to the point that all change stops. Recognizing that others make mistakes and that we can all learn from them is a powerful way of learning. Creating an environment in which mistakes made through genuine effort are recognized, accepted and acted upon is a crucial part of the change process. We must learn to recognize that trying to make

---

Practice point
Always review changes
Allow changes to settle

Practice point
Mistakes should be:
- recognized
- accepted
- acted upon

change will lead to some mistakes if we are to be successful in managing continuous change.

So, a simple process, that is all too difficult to put into practice. This process, by the way, can be used in big organizations and small organizations, and at every level. The only thing that changes is the timescale and complexity of working with greater numbers of people. I and many others have tried it, and it does work, but it is not easy.

CHANGING THE CULTURE

Organizations become very set in the way they do things and the way they behave. This is particularly true in the NHS which is based on strong personal values and often has to deal with the most difficult problems in the most difficult circumstances. Yet, too often, the culture of the organization is centred on the institution rather than on the patient. Much change has taken place on this in recent years and there have been huge and successful changes that must continue. Table 12.1 shows where I believe we should move from and where we should move to in managing for change.

Changing culture is the most difficult of all activities. Culture is based on an inherent set of values matched by an ongoing set of activities, often developed over a number of years. But leadership can, and should, be prepared to change the culture where it is getting in the way of achieving appropriate results.

Go back and revisit the value set that your organization uses. Make it explicit. Write it down, check it out and circulate it. Use the explicit value set to help people understand what the organization is trying to achieve and how it will work to achieve it.

In Warwickshire we have recently revisited our mission statement and value set and have published it widely within the organization for discussion. A seminar of some 50 or so

> **Organizations**
> - Set
> - Centred on institutions

> **Quality example**
> Resetting values in Warwickshire

Table 12.1 Moving the culture

From	To
Centres on institution	Centres on patient
Centres on status	Centres on contribution
Centres on processes	Centres on results
Centres on personal reward	Centres on shared rewards

staff from all levels of the organization came together to review the proposals for the statement and were able to make changes to ensure that there was support for what we were doing. Box 12.3 shows the current Mission Statement for Warwickshire Health, which is the commissioning organization for the county. This is shown simply as an example, not

---

Box 12.3 Warwickshire Health mission statement

Warwickshire Health is the joint body formed by Warwickshire Health Authority and Warwickshire Family Health Services Authority to commission health care for the people of the county.

Context
- We are part of the NHS.
- We work within national policies and priorities.
- We extend these by agreeing local strategies, policies and priorities.
- We have to work within the total money available to us each year.

Purpose
We aim to ensure that Warwickshire has the healthiest population in the UK by early in the 21st century by:

- Working together with others
- Promoting health
- Preventing disease
- Ensuring high quality health care is delivered.

Values
We will strive to work within the following framework of values:

- People are paramount:
  our public
  our patients
  healthcare workers
- All types of health care are valued
- We will seek equity of access
- We will work with integrity
- We will work as an effective and efficient public service.

---

because it is better or worse than any other such statement. What is important here is that it is written down and published, and people have been involved in drawing it up and will be involved in modifying it.

Work with people to find ways of putting that value set into practice in such a way that we always centre on the most important person, who for us, of course, is the patient. Only by having a clear and explicit value set can the culture work in such a way as to deliver what we want to deliver in what is a continually changing environment.

PEOPLE

As I said at the start of this chapter, managing change would be easy if it were not for people. But of course we could not deliver our service without people. I hope that it has already been made clear that I firmly believe the only way to manage for change is to manage for people. People are by far the most important part of any organizational equation, and yet too often it is people we forget. I believe people need the following four things to work successfully in an organization:

* clarity of purpose
* motivation
* positive feedback
* praise when it is due.

Again a simple list. Again a list that is incredibly difficult to remember when you are in the 'hurly burly' of work. Yet if people are clear about what is expected of them, have taken part in establishing those parameters, have been motivated towards them, and then get positive feedback and praise when it is due, I have no doubt that we can manage all of the necessary change we could need.

The most under-used words in the managerial vocabulary are 'thank you'. I have never understood why, but it is true I am certain. Too often we take good performance for granted and criticize the occasional poor performance. We have got to change the balance of this.

Now, all people are not perfect and some people will be more inclined to help with the process of change than others. It is particularly important to identify in your organization those people who are helpers and those who are blockers; those people who are going to be champions of the change and those who are simply going to follow; those people who are going to drive the change forward and those who will

> **Practice point**
> Identify the people who are:
> * changers
> * blockers
> * followers

simply be passengers on the journey. What counts in managing for change is not the position of the person in the organization, but the personal skills that person can bring to the change. Most of us will have been involved in change in which the most unlikely champion has emerged in the oddest position. It is certainly not always the doctor, ward sister or manager who is the real champion of change, and we must be conscious that we should look in rather different ways at the people in our organizations if we are to find the true champions and drivers who will make change happen effectively. The real leader will, of course, use all of the skills available and not just the most obvious ones.

So often making change is about building relationships. It is about:

- a common set of values
- common objectives
- doing things together
- making mistakes together and learning from them
- sharing problems as well as certainties
- talking **with** each other and not **about** each other
- learning together
- achieving success and building on it.

If we can continually build relationships on this foundation and not just expect them to develop at the point at which we are trying to make change, we will surely find that change is easier to manage and people both get more from work and give more to it.

CONCLUSION

Managing for change is not easy. It is the biggest challenge for leadership at all levels. But we do have to recognize that there are some things, often things that are important to us, that we cannot change. I have a prayer on my office wall which I look at to remind me of this important fact. It says:

> God, grant me the serenity
> to accept the things I cannot change;
> the courage to change the things I can;
> and the wisdom to know the difference.

Important and so true.

Managing for change is going to be essential in what is a continually changing world. If we are to provide excellence in care we have to recognize that we will only do so through people. The people who are our patients, the people who work with us, and the people who are going to lead and manage change. At the end of the day, we must remember that for those of us in the business of caring for people of whatever age, it is the patient who is paramount. If we remember that, and centre everything we do and everything we try to achieve around it, we can certainly manage for change which delivers excellent care.

FURTHER READING

Byham, W.C. (1993) *Zapp! Empowerment in Health Care*, Fawcett Columbine, New York.

Edwards, B. (1993) *The National Health Service – A Manager's Tale*, Nuffield Provincial Hospitals Trust, London.

Humble, J.W. (1970) *Management by Objectives in Action*, McGraw-Hill, London.

Robson, M. (1982) *Quality Circles, A Practical Guide*, Gower, London.

Toffler, A. (1985) *The Adaptive Corporation*, Gower, London.

Developing organizations for quality

13

Tom Keighley

EDITORS' INTRODUCTION

The previous chapter looked in detail at different approaches to quality systems and identified common themes among the quality professionals with a strong emphasis on people. These areas are again emphasized in Chapter 13.

It looks at factors that enhance or inhibit good quality organizational change. It discusses how many recent changes have provided disincentives, diminished the value of professional standards of care and moved the care of elderly people from expert to non-expert hands with the transfer of cost from health care to private individuals.

It emphasizes the need for a corporate approach with good and repeated communications with a central focus on the professional voice and consumer. GP fundholders are highlighted as defining simple, practical, measurable standards that directly relate to patient care. It suggests that health commissioners often do not get adequate advice on consumer wishes or professional views.

Key topics
- Introduction
- Selected approaches
- Focus on care of elderly people

The first Griffiths Report (DHSS, 1983) could be read as having two themes: accountability and quality. The report makes a good place to start the consideration of developing organizations for quality because the last decade has been an era of unprecedented organizational change. The health service has seen new structures created and implemented,

Unprecedented organizational change
- Record levels of demoralization
- New thinking about care of elderly people
- Capped budgets
- Patient forms

Quality Care for Elderly People. Edited by Peter P. Mayer, Edward J. Dickinson and Martin Sandler. Published in 1997 by Chapman & Hall, London. ISBN 0 412 61830 3

new processes of care developed and new forms of education for health care professionals introduced. The notion of a market in health care has emerged, as has the concept of evidence-based health care delivery. The impact of this on staff has been profound. Record levels of demoralization, and even a marked increase in the incidence of suicide have been reported among health care professionals.

This has been a period of change akin to the major movement of a tectonic plate. For many, the analogy is a good one because as the new National Health Service (NHS) emerges, it is like the continents drifting apart to form still ill-discerned land masses. It is a period of uncertainty for many in the NHS, an uncertainty fed by constant change in role, function and structure.

Parallel to this reformulation of the NHS, there emerged new thinking and new practices in caring for elderly people. Characterized in different ways, it was described as 'care in the community' and was part of a process to deinstitutionalize the care of elderly people, to give the prime responsibility for their care to local authorities, and to encourage the independent sector to develop and provide non-hospital-based institutional care. With this client group, as with the rest of the NHS, patterns of education and training changed and, as the average age of admission to medical and surgical facilities advanced to over 65 years, the geriatricians became 'physicians of elderly care' and moved from the back wards of the hospitals to centre stage.

Finally, the third major element of change came into play: budgets were capped. The era of financial expansion came to an end for managers and health care professionals alike. The need to work within limited resources, to give an account of their use and be prepared to debate the efficacy and economics of health care delivery has been a difficult pill to swallow. The more open-minded have seen this as an era when new managerial skills have had to be learnt. However, many have observed that while the machinery has been put into place to make doctors and nurses more accountable to non-clinical managers, the accountability of the organizations they work in has been centralized and become less democratic. This change has been delivered in parallel with a new focus on the patient as consumer. *The Patient's Charter* (DoH, 1995) and the hospital league tables are an attempt to make health services more responsive, but the resource capping and politicization of health care has made the change feel like a double-bind: the service must be more responsive to users and cost less, but at the same time the service will be exposed to media-wide criticism and comment. For health care professionals and for managers these are difficult things to achieve. Developing organizations for quality has often been a positive way through this.

SELECTED APPROACHES TO DEVELOPING ORGANIZATIONS FOR QUALITY

Whenever two 'quality gurus' meet to discuss quality, a new quality system emerges! To add to the confusion, the systems have odd acronyms, e.g. CQI, TQM, or paradoxical names which flatter to deceive, e.g. learning organizations or patient-focused hospitals. It is not that these approaches are wrong or irrelevant, but that they and many other developments are faddish. Too often they have just been today's idea or the flavour of the month. Sadly, they are often not related to any form of problem identification in the organizational structure or process, and do not have the clear identifiable outcomes that would achieve long-term commitment to the work involved. However, these weaknesses have not stopped organizations introducing them and committing massive amounts of energy and resources to the work. On occasion, the outcomes seem to have been very positive. However, there is little by way of research to demonstrate this (Attree, 1993).

This lack of evidential base led the Nation Health Service Executive (NHSE) to convene a working group under the heading 'Quality in Action'. Their report (NHSE, 1995), issued prior to the production of a 'toolbox' later in 1995, is useful in identifying the strengths and weaknesses of the current situation. The report recognizes the ideal situation as being one in which:

- a corporate vision and language is shared by all
- a central core set of values exists
- quality is a way of life for everyone within the NHS
- the NHS is a listening organization.

The worst-case scenario is one where:

- quality drops off the agenda
- quality is rejected by the professions
- there is ever-increasing customer dissatisfaction
- no real change occurs

Approaching quality
- Caution with 'systems'
- NHS working party
- Promoting and blocking factors
- Core-factor approach

- there are variations in quality
- the organization is driven by its interest in establishing quality systems rather than being people-driven.

The current situation is identified thus:

- the corporate vision of quality is not central, nor is it shared throughout the NHS
- quality is patchy with some good work being done but also some poor efforts
- there is variable commitment/investment from the boards and senior managers
- some end-users are unable to drive the process of quality improvement.

This set of views is interesting because it offers a semistructured approach to considering why the development of organizations for quality has been such a problem in the NHS. The gap between the ideal and worst cases is immense and is not bridged by the view of the current situation. Indeed, one might well come to the conclusion that the present and worst-case scenarios are uncomfortably close. Indeed, the report goes on to consider this in more detail by identifying the factors that would lead to a more ideal situation (Box 13.1) and those that would be associated with a worst-case scenario (Box 13.2).

Box 13.1   Ideal factors

- Effective corporate leadership
- Standards and shared values
- Credibility with customers
- Customer awareness
- Belief in the quality process
- Investment in people
- Corporate identity
- Politics, the media and charters
- Recruitment, selection and staff development
- Research and development, protocols and standards
- Health of the nation
- Staff empowerment
- Enthusiasm and excitement
- Purchasing leverage

Box 13.2   Worst-case factors

- Resistance to change
- Professional group clashes
- Professional quality versus managerial quality
- Poor communications
- Poor outcome measures
- Quality not integrated in the business plan
- Lack of knowledge and understanding
- Barriers between categories of care
- Fear

The worst-case scenario is one that perhaps has greater resonance in many organizations. The comparison between the two lists is very worrying. Most of all, one is forced to ask how to achieve a move from one scenario to another.

Particularly when considering the care of elderly people, who can be viewed as a group in the community that is especially vulnerable and less able to represent itself, the worst case factors are the ones that could cause major disruption in the care services they are offered. It is therefore important to focus on the core factors that can develop the quality of service being offered. The following list is not new. Anyone who has managed health services will realize that they have been pursuing these issues throughout their time in management positions. When they are demystified, they can be addressed with greater clarity. Demystification also puts the list of ideal and worst-case scenarios into perspective:

1. Focus on the business in hand
2. Employing the best people
3. How we get things done around here
4. Leadership.

These subsume the terms identified above, and when worked on consistently achieve high levels of quality in service delivery.

FOCUS ON THE BUSINESS IN HAND

In times past, this was never a problem for the NHS. It was set up as a crusade to treat the sick and improve the health

---

of the nation. As a public service, it attracted a range of health care professionals and administrators who largely shared a humane belief in the role and function of the NHS.

Griffiths' criticisms of the service alluded to earlier brought to a head a decade of political discontent with the management of the health service. It came as a shock to many health care professionals that there were questions to be asked about the way they delivered care and what the outcomes of that care were. Shaw (1993) points out that the clinical professions responded to this by increasing their determination to maintain standards. He goes on to point out, however, that a third factor came into play – the consumer movement, which was demanding to know much more about public and professional services.

These three changes – which can be summarized as new national NHS initiatives, professional standard setting and consumerism – caused a loss of focus on what the business was. Organizations constructed with quality as their prime focus need an innate understanding of the nature of their business and the demand in the market place that drives it. However, this triad of different foci is the prime reason why a sense of uncertainty has crept into discussions about the business of the health service. The national NHS initiatives (reforms, developments, etc.) all point to the business of the NHS being able to achieve the objectives of the Secretary of State. The epidemic of standard setting in the health care professions suggests that the objective is to improve, maintain and, in some cases, defend professional practice. The emergence of consumerism in the health service has raised serious questions about who the customers are and how they might want to exercise their rights and/or expectations as such. It has become a scenario in which the 'business in hand' is no longer determined by the health care professionals, the patients or the politicians, but by a mediating of all three factors at a local level.

The current material representation of this is the service contract agreed between the commissioner and the provider. Given its importance, it was worrying to see in the then Health Minister Dr Mahwinney's papers at a conference on purchasing in 1994 (NHSE, 1994) that the role of the provider clinician in contract setting was one of the areas of concern. Expert input is clearly central to deciding both the nature of the service to be provided and the criteria by which its success is to be determined. Once this has been achieved, the era of standards, clinical guidelines, protocols, etc. may pass

Three changes
- NHS initiatives
- Professional standard setting
- Consumerism
- The cause and loss of focus

Expert input is essential
- Nature of service
- Criteria
- Informed judgement

away, and an informed judgement may be made about the business in hand based on a debate about clinical judgement and resource availability rather than on a framework in which the commissioner, ill-informed about clinicians and consumer views, seeks to determine contracts on a case-load basis.

To achieve this, greater clarity is required in three ways. First, the commissioners need to take on a much stronger role in informing themselves about patients' wishes to go alongside their health needs assessment work. Second, all health care professions need to sign up to the development of hub and spoke specialisms (Calman, 1994) with a general pursuit of excellence, rather than just a few centres being given the responsibility to be 'leading edge'. Third, the difference between consumers and consumerism must be acted upon. While groups can bring pressure for change, health care delivery is always about the case of one person. Too often, general approaches have focused on the larger group, obscuring the needs of individuals and subgroups. When considering a group like 'the elderly', which is concerned with the provision of services for people from the age of 60 years onwards, the need to appreciate variation in service delivery is acute.

The determination of the business in hand is therefore crucial. Achieving the organizational and individual sophistication to achieve this is often the challenge. The lack of training and education to help everyone concerned understand this, is one of the reasons that the focus has been lost. The other is a degree of alienation induced by the nature of the changes being pursued in the NHS. Perhaps this is inevitable, but failure to address it will only lead to evermore people deciding to pursue their own agendas. This takes the focus off the business in hand and undermines the quality of service in the organization. This dysfunctional activity is organizational bad news, and leads to the next point.

Quality needs
- Commisioners informed of patients' wishes
- General pursuit of excellence
- Act on the difference between consumers and consumerism

EMPLOYING THE BEST PEOPLE

Once the focus on the business in hand is clear, the next stage is to employ the best people to deliver that business. This used to be, and occasionally can still be found to be, the case in the NHS. The great threat to the quality of care delivery comes from the deconstruction of roles and services. This refers to the process by which care facilities for elderly peo-

Current threat-transfer of care
- to different sectors
- to different staff

ple have been moved from hospitals to local authorities and the independent sector. This has occurred in parallel with major changes in staffing structures.

A paradox has been played out in both of these changes. The first is that the rationale for moving people from hospitals into local authority care was to keep them in their community and prevent illness or ageing being the determining factor in how elderly people lived their lives. Mitchell, Kafetz and Rossiter (1987), among others, described how and why this could be done. However, it obscured the fact that for many elderly people, the lack of hospital accommodation is resulting in inappropriate placement for their continuing care, and that the cost of care in the community was likely to be higher when fully costed than the cost of care in hospitals. It is likely that the real saving here is achieved by transferring the cost from the health service to the private purse of individuals or their relatives (Nitjkamp *et al.*, 1991).

The second paradox here is that the transfer has been associated with a transfer from expert carers to untrained carers. Ironically, the care of elderly people in hospital has become a specialty whose time has come, and instead of being seen as the 'Cinderella' service, it is increasingly becoming an area of practice that is viewed as complex, valued and highly regarded. The number of specialist programmes for NHS carers (doctors, nurses and professions allied to medicine) all point to the way in which it has become a more highly valued area of work. In contrast, elderly people are often being discharged to local authority accommodation, nursing homes or their own homes, where the direct care is to be delivered by individuals who have had little or no preparation. This shift was compounded by some of the education reforms in nursing (UKCC, 1986), under which student nurses were replaced by care assistants, so that the number of staff available for employment in the independent sector was constrained. The central role of the NHS as a trainer of care staff for the independent sector and, to a certain degree, for the local authorities, has not been appreciated.

Getting the best staff is central to any strategy for service delivery; this process of change has undermined that. However, the increase in the provision of specialist development opportunities in the NHS has heralded an era of role extension for many health care professionals engaged in caring for elderly people. The need for greater expertise is probably going to increase. However, employing the best people goes hand in hand with keeping them. Ironically, that is best achieved not by offering high salaries (though that is always highly appreciated!), but by the provision of development opportunities and an environment that is supportive, encouraging and valuing of the work being undertaken.

In developing organizations for quality, getting good staff is one thing, developing them to respond positively to the changes and demands of the reforming NHS is another. In a review of the development of auditing in nursing care, Balogh (1992) was able to demonstrate strong links between the quality of care given and the labour force issues. The need to address this is central to any strategy aimed at delivering good quality care, and is directly tied to the next issue.

HOW WE GET THINGS DONE AROUND HERE

This phrase is an excellent and straightforward definition of the term organizational culture. This is a complex issue and has been addressed in detail in other publications (Keighley, 1993). Its centrality to the development of an organization, let alone any judgement about quality in an organization, should not be ignored. The sources of organizational culture are often obscure and varied. However, some components can be assessed and influenced. Training and education are key determinants of culture, as are peer pressure and social expectation.

> **Determinants of culture**
> - Training and education
> - Peer pressure
> - Social expectations

These three elements are all open to influence, but in different ways. The lack of influence on the education and training provided to health care professionals by practitioners and managers can partly explain the mismatch in culture that occurs between trainees and practitioners. Closer working relationships between the education providers and education commissioners will emerge as a result of the restructuring of the regional function. It will make it the direct responsibility of the service providers to commission the education and training they require within the framework of Working Paper 10 (DoH, 1989). Clearly, educators will need to be able to demonstrate their responsiveness to the needs of the service. Equally, the service providers will have to take responsibility for better definition of the nature of the individual they want to emerge from the education process.

One problem here is that medical education and medical appointments still sit very tightly within the framework of the medical schools and medical royal colleges. This is currently a source of concern in the NHS because of the difficulties it causes in making appointments. When considering the care of elderly people, the education and appointment process has also to be seen from the point of view of availability and flexibility. Producing health care professionals who cannot/will not be responsive to the changes in service delivery and service profile will not produce a culture that fits with the expectations of the service.

Two other elements that determine organizational culture are peer pressure and social expectation. One factor that has influenced both of these, and will become an increasing influence, is the use of audit and other outcome-based processes to influence performance. Roberts, Khee and Philp (1994) demonstrated high levels of agreement among geriatricians in their study on performance measures for geriatric services. The authors compared the views of the doctors with the opinions of the patients. While there was much overlap, there was also marked disagreement, and the authors point to the need for more than one group to be engaged in the discussion.

Philp *et al.* (1994), from the same team at Southampton, looked at participatory ways to introduce change. One of the findings of the study was that only one group of staff was able to change its practice: nurses. This demonstrates vividly the difficulty faced. Achieving change is complex, and if it runs counter to 'the way we get things done around here', it will be more difficult still. One of the major positives in such a situation is the nature of the leadership.

LEADERSHIP

Nearly every author who has written on the subject of quality has talked about the need for leadership, and usually leadership from 'the top'. It is one of those strange phenomena of the modern UK public sector that the leadership at the top of organizations is both more visible and yet more diffuse.

The creation of a chief executive model of working has in theory established a clear leadership position at the top of the organization. How that leadership is exercised is another matter. For many, it is a 'buck stops here' type of position and has become a defensive, back-room function with the more public role being taken by the chairman or chairwoman of the organization. Too often this is a good guy/bad guy act with the chairman/chairwoman promoting the positive developments and the good news, while the chief executive is left to do the public sweeping up. To develop an organization for quality, it is imperative that the leadership function in the organization is clear at every level. This is achievable in the health care arena because the system is essentially hierarchical. Fortunately, much of the status differentiation is being lost as effective teams come into existence, but the hierarchical reporting structure does mean that it is possible to identify functional areas and levels.

The problem that has occurred with quality, however, is that leadership has so often not come from 'the top'. Too often, the quality brief has been vested elsewhere on the board and has been espoused by enthusiasts and change agents in the system. As a result, as indicated earlier, different types of quality initiatives have emerged and have occasionally been in conflict.

Many health care professionals have been offended by a focus on quality that ignored the fact that every element of their professional education and development had been aimed at producing a high quality practitioner. This has been underpinned by the confetti cloud of standards and guidelines that have emerged in the last decade. In parallel with this, the quality enthusiasts have been focusing on other items that health care professionals have not always rated as significant. For example, a consultant who has saved the life of a trauma victim is not usually impressed if a full scale investigation is launched when the patient complains of a skin reaction to the adhesive tape! The failure to draw together the two perspectives on quality is usually evidence that the quality exercise is not being led from the top.

It is the function of the chief executive to get ownership for the work of developing a quality organization. The senior staff in the different parts of the organization have an equal responsibility to achieve that integration of purpose and activity in their own part of the organization. The need to speak with one voice through the organization is the practical representation of leadership. This should be matched by a willingness to repeat the same message continuously.

One of the amazing elements in the experience of leadership is the forgetfulness and ability to misinterpret or reinterpret otherwise clear and simple messages that occurs with colleagues. It is a reflection of the cultural issues touched on earlier, and an indication of the importance of good and simple communication. To create and deliver a quality

> **Quality**
> - Should be led from the top
> - Should recognize professional standards
> - Should not trivialize

> **Practice point**
> - One voice
> - Repeat messages
> - Good and simple communication

organization the most important function of leading is to ensure clear messages are given but also that responses are heard and understood. This underpins the development of the quality organization more effectively than any concern about structure, process or outcome. In the modern organization all of these can change. If the communication is effective, it can all be managed in a comparatively straightforward manner.

FOCUS ON CARE OF ELDERLY PEOPLE

In concluding this chapter it is appropriate to highlight some issues that are particularly pertinent to the development of organizations for quality when that organization is dedicated to the care of elderly people. Not only is this an expanding group in the population, its structure in terms of age, social status, political clout and economic power will change significantly after the turn of the century. Already, elderly people are developing the means to represent themselves and their wishes much more extensively. The need for health services to be aware of this and to respond to it is long overdue. This will be a feature of how GP fundholders exercise their role in relation to their elderly patients, acting as advocates and advisers to support them and guide them through the intricacies of the three service divisions; NHS, local authorities and the independent sector. The views of GP fundholders about quality is proving to be remarkably uncomplicated. They want assurances about who will see their patient, that there will be little or no waiting times and that there will be no unwanted complications to deal with after discharge, e.g. infections or pressure sores. Equally, they are expecting carers to be expert and relevant; so if a patient is admitted for medical or surgical interventions they expect the consultant and nursing team to be skilled in the treatment and care of elderly people. One might conclude that these are not exceptional expectations, but they cannot be met everywhere.

A second issue is how the workforce available to care for elderly people is going to change. Nitjkamp and colleagues (1991) pointed out that across Europe the population is ageing as the birthrate falls: the consequence of this is that in the future there will be fewer people to deliver care and fewer people to be taxed or to contribute to insurance schemes to fund the care. This means that as the next century

GP fundholders
- Advocates and advisers
- Have simple quality standards

progresses, people can expect to have to pay more for the care they receive and the nature of that care will change as there are fewer people to deliver it. There are, of course, many consequences of this, but as regards the development of organizations and other forms of services, there will need to be a dramatic rethink about their form and the judgements made about their adequacy.

Finally, a thought about the ethics of caring for elderly people in the light of this scenario. With resources constrained by a diminishing population, and yet ever greater and more extensive therapies available for treating elderly people, it is very likely that the quality of care offered to elderly people will be challenged by the resource-generating part of the population. To prevent the negative consequences of this and to address it positively, there is a need to have a public- and society-wide debate that goes far beyond the sniping currently underway about local authority resourcing. The implications of this are too great to be left to politicians.

REFERENCES

Attree, M. (1993) An analysis of the concept of 'quality' as it relates to contemporary nursing care. *International Journal of Nursing Studies*, 30(4), 355–69.

Balogh, R. (1992) Audits of nursing care in Britain: a review and a critique of approaches to validating them. *International Journal of Nursing Studies*, 29(2), 119–33.

Calman, K. (1994) *A policy framework for commissioning cancer services: Report of the Expert Advisory Group to the Chief Medical Officer for England and Wales*, HMSO, London.

Department of Health (1989) *Working for Patients: Education and Training. Working Paper 10*, HMSO, London.

Department of Health (1995) *The Patient's Charter and You*, HMSO, London.

Department of Health and Social Security (1983) *Recommendations on the effective use of manpower and related resources. Report of the NHS Management Inquiry Team (The Griffiths Report)*, HMSO, London.

Keighley, T. (1993). Managing health care delivery, in *Nursing practice and health care*, 2nd edn [eds S. Hinchliff, S.E. Norman and J.E. Schober), Edward Arnold, London, pp. 266–99.

Mitchell, J., Kafetz, K. and Rossiter, B. (1987) Benefits of effective hospital services for elderly people. *British Medical Journal*, **295**, 980–4.

NHS Executive (1994) *Involving local people: purchasing for health: A speech by Dr Brian Mawhinney MP, Minister for Health,*

National Purchasing Conference, Birmingham, 13 April 1994, Department of Health, Leeds.

NHS Executive (1995) *Quality in action: a focus on quality. A report on the outcomes of three Focus on Quality workshops. Sponsored by the NHS Executive between July 1993 and March 1994*, Department of Health, Leeds.

Nitjkamp, P., Pacolet, J., Spinnewyn, H. *et al.* (1991) *National diversity and European trends in services for the elderly*, University of Leuven, Higher Institute of Labour Studies, Leuven, Belgium.

Philp, I., Goddard, A., Connell, N.A. *et al.* (1994) Development and evaluation of an information system for quality assurance. *Age and Ageing*, **23**(2), 150–3.

Roberts, H., Khee, T.S. and Philp, I. (1994) Setting priorities for measures of performance for geriatric medical services. *Age and Ageing*, **23**(2), 154–7.

Shaw, C.D. (1993) Quality assurance in the United Kingdom. *Quality Assurance in Health Care*, **5**(2), 107–18.

United Kingdom Central Council for Nursing, Midwifery and Health Visiting (1986) *Project 2000: a new preparation for practice*, UKCC, London.

The future care of elderly people

14

Elizabeth M. Smith and
Peter H. Millard

EDITORS' INTRODUCTION

The last chapter in the book presents the perceptions of a trainee and a professor of geriatric medicine who was president of the British Geriatrics Society. This provides a comprehensive account of the major features of the specialty and the needs of its patients with a special emphasis on mathematical modelling for the management of services; the centrality of long-term care and its control are also considered.

It proposes that appropriately timed assessments of the needs of elderly people by the multidisciplinary team will avoid hospital admission and prevent long-term institutional care. The need for care is not infinite and it is feasible to remove waiting lists and to control the requirement for long-term care. The chapter argues that control of the latter sector is essential to provide an effective care service for elderly people.

It goes further, to suggest that the size of the long-term care sector determines the size and activity of other health care sectors. It shows that data that are readily available through hospital administration systems can be used as the basis for the calculations needed. The authors state that controlled discharge and the threshold of non-discharge are further crucial elements.

The final section looks at strategies of care, varying from preventive and health promotion approaches, through education and assessment, to the development of specific services to reduce the requirement for long-term institutional care.

Key topics
- Basic principles
- Central place of long-term care
- A model for designing care
- Action to support the long-term care approach
- Quality in long-term care

Quality Care for Elderly People. Edited by Peter P. Mayer, Edward J. Dickinson and Martin Sandler. Published in 1997 by Chapman & Hall, London. ISBN 0 412 61830 3

> There is a clear message that moving people to services increases mortality and no future planner of services for elderly people should see progressive care, whether in housing, institutions or hospitals, as necessarily the best model for the care of elderly people.

INTRODUCTION

Three approaches
- Foster dependency
- Do nothing
- Active approach

During the next decade the number of older people in the world population will increase rapidly, while the relative proportion of younger people participating in the workforce will decline. Accordingly, the problem of caring for frail or sick elderly people requires urgent attention, particularly in Western countries where there is an environment of economic recession and government cut-backs in health and social welfare. There are three possible approaches: foster dependency; do nothing; or encourage an active, therapeutic, knowledge-based, multidisciplinary approach. Only by taking such an approach will the world come to terms with the success of ageing and avoid inappropriately high levels of long-term institutional care.

As the problem is new, new strategic approaches are needed. Because disease presents differently in elderly people, and multiple pathology is the exception not the rule, local strategies based on single diseases, denial of admission and rapid early discharge must be modified. Key facts that necessitate a change in policy are that many people over the age of 80 years live alone, are often subnourished, disabled and reliant on formal and informal networks of care. To succeed, the threshold for admission to hospital needs to be lower, while the threshold for discharge needs to be higher. This does not imply that elderly people should be permanently institutionalized, far from it; rather it implies that an active, properly staffed and equipped hospital department specializing in the optimistic management of elderly people is the key to success.

Many people over 80
- live alone
- are subnourished
- are disabled
- are reliant on care

The majority of elderly people can be rehabilitated to successful independent living at home. However, correct management takes time, and doctors in all specialties must ensure that elderly people are fit to return home. The active management of elderly people requires skilled medical, nursing, therapy and social work care and a changed environment. The UK led the world in the introduction of an acute therapeutic approach to the management of disability in old age and some countries are following this lead. This is the correct approach. Most other countries tackle the problem of dependency in old age in a negative way.

In the UK, the House of Lords Working Party on Medical Ethics recently decided that introducing euthanasia was not in the interests of our population (House of Lords, 1994). We agree. Where there are excellent hospices, well developed community services and active departments of geriatric medicine staffed by physicians with special responsibility for the medical management of elderly people, a country does not need to foster euthanasia. Governments throughout the world need to recognize the benefits to be gained from introducing physician-led rehabilitation into the medical and social management of elderly people. Defining medical responsibility, not interest, is the key to the development of geriatric medical services (Warren, 1943; Millard, 1991a).

In the past 50 years a knowledge base concerning the complex problems of the medical, social and psychological management of elderly people has been identified. Starting from the attack on bed-rest, new skills have been identified relating to the management of illness. Central to any global strategy for the management of ageing has to be the identification and dissemination of the entirely new knowledge base of geriatric medicine and gerontology. To succeed, countries throughout the world must modify the way that they train their doctors, nurses, therapy staff and social workers. Understanding and controlling resource use is fundamental to the development of health care systems for an ageing population.

> **Practice point**
> Understanding and controlling resource use is fundamental

This chapter discusses the basic principles that are involved and outlines possible ways forward. Each country has to decide how best to provide services for its ageing population within the limits of its available resources. All over the world decision makers have to make choices. Unlike in the USA, the question in the UK is not 'should there be a National Health Service?'; rather the question is 'what place should hospitals play in the community care of an ageing population?' We argue that the correct way forward is to develop combined hospital- and community-based social and medical services for the total care of elderly people in the 21st century.

BASIC PRINCIPLES

Ethical principles

The medical and social problems of elderly people are complex. They involve social, psychological, biological and environmental components that physicians cannot solve alone. In managing illness in old age, doctors need to balance enthusiasm with the realization that death is part of life. Three fundamental ethical principles should underpin our decision making process.

1. The inviolability of life: physicians must not kill patients either by acts of commission or acts of omission.
2. The finite nature of life: physicians and their teams should not strive officiously to keep alive patients whose death is clearly inevitable.
3. The need for equity: any treatment given to an elderly person should reflect the current, peer reviewed, normative values concerning the correctness of treatment.

Service principles

Given that a society accepts the ethical principles listed above, then three service principles follow.

1. The community, as well as the family, has a duty to care. Families, neighbours and volunteers provide the informal network, while health and social services provide the formal network. Each has to provide services 24 hours a day. To run community services, hospital departments of geriatric medicine must have empty beds.
2. Professionals have a duty to see that the assets of the community and the family are used wisely and well. Saving money in hospital by forcing either the family or the community to spend more money on care is not in the interests of either party. Consequently, national and local services must be based on concepts of public rather than private economics.
3. Informal care must be given by trained staff. Value for money, equity and justice, implies that all staff caring for elderly people in hospital and the community must be properly trained and supplied with adequate equipment to do their work.

Operational principles

In 1985 in the *Journal of the American Geriatrics Society*, Pfeiffer suggested some basic principles to consider when dealing with elderly people (Pfeiffer, 1985). The eight principles make an excellent starting point.

1. Older patients are treatable.
2. Care of the elderly requires a multidisciplinary approach.
3. Intervention in the life of an older person should always be preceded by a comprehensive assessment of that patient's overall functioning.
4. Care of the elderly requires a new kind of service: co-ordination of services or case management.
5. The role of the family is critically important in the treatment of older patients.
6. Care of the elderly requires special training in geriatrics and gerontology.
7. Not only are older patients treatable, they are teachable.
8. Older patients are not only treatable, they are teachable, they also teach us about old age.

> **Practice point**
> Principles of excellent care

These principles are based on the fact that disease presents differently in old age and often comes disguised as social problems. Falling, inability to cope, immobility or confusion are symptoms of disease, not age.

Therefore, no one should be admitted to permanent care without preadmission, multidisciplinary assessment and in-patient rehabilitation.

> **Practice point – to avoid long-term care**
> • Preadmission assessment
> • Multidisciplinary assessment
> • Inpatient rehabilitation

A TOTAL SERVICE

In 1943 Warren proposed the development of geriatrics as a specialty within medicine (Warren, 1943). In the following summary of her paper, Millard has changed the words chronic sick to aged (Millard, 1991a).

1. A higher standard and a great deal more work is needed in the care of the aged.
2. The aged should be diagnosed and treated in special blocks in the general hospital set up that are equipped for the purpose.
3. The aged should be admitted to homes through hospital units only. All homes should be attached to hospital units to ensure close follow-up.

It is to be hoped that the 21st century will see these policies being implemented, for all countries need to find better, more efficient, ways of caring for elderly people in their society. Underlying different views of how this should be done is the recognition that in so doing we will be taking responsibility for ourselves. We should all ask ourselves how we want to be living 40, 30, 20, 10 or five years from now. Given the choice, would you prefer a fragmented or a co-ordinated service?

The central place of long-term care

Multidisciplinary physician-led rehabilitation is central to the control of health care resources at any age (Warren, 1943). Proper assessment, accurate diagnosis and correct treatment in a changed environment is essential (Horrocks, 1986): without this the number of people in care just expands to fill the resources that are provided. Contrary to current economic thinking, the demand for health care is not infinite. In any catchment area the number of people aged over 65 years is a finite number; at the very most the number in care can only expand to reach the total number of elderly people in the catchment area. Start from that point and you can begin to plan rationally.

Questions to be asked are:

- How many older people live in the catchment area?
- How many hospital, rest and nursing home places are available?
- How many residents, clients or patients were admitted permanently in the preceding 12 months?
- How many people will you want to admit permanently in the next year?
- How many beds do you want to make available for admission and respite care?

Quality example
How to get rid of the waiting list

For example, in 1976 the London Borough of Merton had 300 residential places and a waiting list for admission to the homes of 160. The previous year, only 90 people were admitted. Clearly, in 1977, unless there was an epidemic of influenza, the waiting list would never be cleared and at least 70 people would be disappointed. So the borough decided to scrap the waiting list, convert one 30-bedded home to respite care, and introduce preadmission multidisciplinary assessment prior to residential home admission.

Table 14.1 explains why it is important to control long-term care. The table shows that controlling long-term care is

Table 14.1 Acute, rehabilitation and long stay: incidence and prevalence

Yearly incidence	Average daily prevalence	Cost per year at £300 per week (£)
25 cases per year staying two weeks	1	15 600
25 cases per year staying three months	6	93 600
25 cases per year staying four years	100	1 560 000

simply a matter of understanding the difference between incidence and prevalence. Note that 25 people rehabilitated over three months at £300 a week cost £93 600 a year, while 25 people not rehabilitated cost £1 560 000 a year. That is why expenditure on medical leadership of multidisciplinary management in long-term care is the most cost-efficient use of resources (Millard, 1991a).

A MODELLING APPROACH

In collaboration with computer scientists, operational researchers and mathematicians, we are developing a modelling approach to the planning of health care systems (Harrison and Millard, 1991; Millard and McClean, 1994, 1996). Such models may assist decision makers who do not then need to experiment in the real world. Explanatory models will assist in care system development, as have models of organ systems in the past.

The model has several advantages (McClean, 1994). Readily available data is used, e.g. the midnight bed state. It explains behaviour in terms that are plausible to professionals and mathematically credible (Harrison and Millard, 1991; McClean and Millard, 1993; Irvine, McClean and Millard, 1994). The model may provide a useful tool for planning future services (Case study 14.1).

Mixed exponential model uses
- readily available data
- is explanatory
- credible

Case study 14.1 Resource use by flow

Modelling
It can be shown that different wards and services have different rates of flow (Millard, 1992). In every ward the rate of

flow represents the interaction of staff, patients and resources (Feldstein, 1964), and the prevailing behaviour represents past training and current decision making.

Changing resources without changing knowledge does not, per se, introduce changed behaviour, but when behaviour changes the rate of flow changes from constant to constant (Millard, 1992). Under pressure, staff alter admission rather than change discharge behaviour.

Thus long-stay patient numbers can rise and fall independently of age changes in the community (Millard, 1992). Since there is marked variation internationally in the allocation of resources to long-term care (Grundy and Arie, 1984), the number in care is independent of age.

Long-stay bed availability occurs mainly through death, with discharge rare after 90 days of admission (Silver and Zuberi, 1965), but admissions rise when long-stay beds are designated for rehabilitation and vice versa (Millard, 1992).

Exponential analysis identifies resource utilization compartments and flow rate components of bed occupancy, while bed occupancy measures alone confuse bed occupancy and use (Yates, 1982).

Table 14.2 shows that the key component is the control of long-term care, and that if overall resources are fixed, increasing the proportion of long-stay beds increases the number of people treated.

Table 14.2 Impact of changing the balance of short- and long-stay patients within a department of geriatric medicine*

			Admissions		
Allocated beds	*Number short- stay*	*Number long- stay*	*Short stay[†] ×12*	*Long stay[‡] ×0.5*	*Total*
100	20	80	240	40	280
100	40	60	480	30	510
100	60	40	720	20	740
100	80	20	960	10	970

*First published in the *Journal of the Royal Society of Medicine* (1991), **84**, 732. Reproduced with permission.
[†]Assuming 12 admissions per acute bed per year, i.e. an average flow rate of 36 days.
[‡]Assuming 0.5 admissions per long-stay bed per year, i.e. an average flow rate of 2 years.

In addition, resource availability in the community influences patient flows. Short-stay turnover is greatest where discharge to institutional care is easy and access to rehabilitation poor (Millard, 1994). Both the local availability of nursing home and community care services will affect outcomes.

The model shows that it is essential to control entry to long-term care, whether by peer review (Millard, 1989), or through assessment criteria implemented in the UK in April, 1996.

Spending time to reduce levels of disability is a better use of resources than increasing rapidity of throughput with poor outcomes. This model can be used in a variety of settings and takes into account patient flow and compartmental thresholds. A software package is available. (St George's Hospital Medical School http://www.sghms.ac.uk)

What if?

The most important question that clinicians and managers have to answer is: 'what will happen if I change bed numbers, or alter the way patients are treated?' The benefit to be gained from flow rate modelling is that hypothetical questions like this one can be pretested. Using flow rate models, it rapidly becomes apparent that the key to the provision of health care is the control of entry into long-term care in hospital or in the community (Warren, 1943; Millard, 1991a; Harrison and Millard, 1991).

When medically-led, knowledge-based, active, purposeful, multidisciplinary rehabilitation is not provided in purpose-designed environments, long-term patient numbers increase, they block beds and consume resources that could be used for others. Contrary to popular belief, the correct approach is to admit potential long-stay patients early (Hodkinson and Jeffreys, 1972) rather than deny them access to hospitals, because with enablement and supportive postdischarge care, the majority can be enabled to lead full lives within the limits of their disability. Therefore, to provide health care all we need is a few long-stay beds protected by many active beds (Bagnall *et al.*, 1973), rather than many long-stay beds protected by a few acute beds. In other words, to succeed in the management of an ageing population one has to reverse current policies.

> **Practice point**
> - Admit early
> - Aim for few long-term care beds protected by many active beds

ACTION TO SUPPORT THIS LONG-TERM CARE STRATEGY

This section looks at the actions needed to ensure an active, high quality and cost-effective service.

Health promotion

The three most important aspects of health promotion are good diet, regular exercise and cessation of smoking.

Adequate income is required to provide for basic needs such as good food, heating and clothing, and to maintain health and prevent morbidity.

At all ages it is essential to provide all the elements for adequate nutrition in a balanced diet that includes fibre in the form of suitable carbohydrates, good quality protein, vitamins and trace elements, fruit and vegetables, adequate calcium, and an avoidance of excess fat. The observed immune decline in old age is probably nutritional (Roebothan and Chandra, 1994).

The importance of vitamin C in tissue healing, bone formation and leucocyte function, and the consequences of a deficiency, mean that supplementation for elder people should be routine. Western institutionalized and housebound people require daily supplementation with 1.2 g of calcium and 800 IU of vitamin D (Chapuy *et al.*, 1992) and 60 mg of vitamin C.

Poverty fosters morbidity and fuels demands for long-term care. Ultimately, if we neglect to provide poor elderly people with an adequate basic income we and the rest of society lose out because we then have to fund health and social care for the ensuing disease and disability.

Exercise

Exercise can help prevent conditions such as osteoporosis and cardiovascular disease, and exercise can help preserve function even when older people are frail (McMurdo and Rennie, 1993). Information is needed on appropriate types of exercise, how long to pursue the activity, and any precautions to take. Use of different types of media with acceptable imagery for elderly people is now being produced.

Local government needs to encourage activities such as cycling by improving cycle lanes in roads. Sports centre swimming pools could provide more designated sessions for

Practice point
Good health requires:
- adequate income
- adequate nutrition

Practice point
- Good diet
- Regular exercise
- Stop smoking

older participants. A more positive portrayal of elderly people in the arts, particularly television and films, may help overcome the natural reticence some elderly people have towards exercise. In the next century we expect that the majority of residents in residential homes, sheltered accommodation and nursing homes will take part in exercise and activity groups.

Smoking cessation

Initiatives to help elderly people stop smoking should include information about the immediate benefit because many elderly people feel they have probably already done the damage and that they might as well continue.

Reducing disability

Deteriorating health is not a normal part of ageing. Increasing dependence always has an underlying medical, social or psychological cause that may be remediable. Elderly people usually consult doctors about medical symptoms such as breathlessness, ankle swelling, weight loss, change in bowel habit, etc. They may not, however, consult for a more subtle deterioration, such as increased difficulty getting out of a chair or climbing stairs. Disability is accepted by elderly people and their families as being inevitable, and poorly trained doctors often reinforce this negative view. A central platform for true success is the education of medical practitioners and care staff about the importance of disability (Case study 14.2).

Case study 14.2   Health checks

In 1990 the UK Government introduced annual primary care health checks for patients aged over 75 years. These provide an opportunity to assess changes in health status (MacLennan, 1990). Not surprisingly, the yield of new problems discovered lessens with each annual visit. This indicates the success of the programme and is not an indication to discontinue, but it may suggest that annual intervals are too frequent. A screening programme performed by trained lay volunteers has been shown to reduce the number of days spent in institutional care but to increase the referral rate to hospital-based services (Carpenter and Demopoulos, 1990). Future investment in health care needs to concentrate on detecting and treating problems at an early stage, in order

> **Practice point**
> Early detection reduces long-term costs

to reduce the costs of the long-term care of dependent people.

To introduce a therapeutic approach to disability, future care systems for elderly people must include properly organized physician-led multidisciplinary assessment.

This is particularly important prior to admission to residential or nursing homes and before packages of care are instituted by social workers in the community. The exact location and position of such multidisciplinary teams may need to vary according to local needs. We think that they should be hospital-based and supported by acute admission beds, day hospitals and respite facilities. Hospital-based teams should also be responsible for the maintenance and supervision of health care in the institutional setting (Warren, 1943; Millard, 1991a).

Acute care

Moving elderly patients produces an increase in mortality, and frail elderly people may become confused when moved to a strange environment, yet it is important not to underestimate the benefit of timely admission to properly staffed and designated wards. As more short-term medical and nursing care becomes available in the community, some acute illnesses can be managed there, but they must be monitored on a daily basis. If the patient is deteriorating, and death is not an expected or inevitable outcome, then the patient should be moved to hospital because delay in admission blunts the clinical effectiveness (Hodkinson and Jeffreys, 1972). This should be supervised by medical specialists (Royal College of Physicians of London, 1994). In future we support the vision of first line admitting physicians with acute and holistic skills supported by specialist physicians (Grimley-Evans, 1994). The central core of this must be a triage system under which patients are assessed and admitted to the place best suited to their needs (Figure 14.1).

All elderly patients in acute hospitals should be assessed by a geriatrician if there has been a change in their disability level. Reassessment should include a secondary clerking in the postacute phase of the admission and examination of cognition, hearing, vision, mobility, and social and environmental needs.

The key to restoring people to the 'well' part of Figure 14.1 is accurate diagnosis, treatment and rehabilitation. Rarely is it possible to achieve this in the community.

Practice point
Moving people may increase mortality

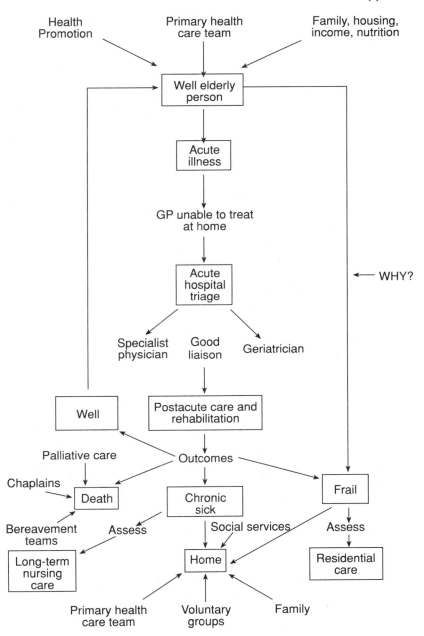

Figure 14.1 A triage system

SPECIFIC SERVICES FOR KEY CONDITIONS – 'THE GERIATRIC GIANTS'

Depression and dementia

Integration between the geriatric and psychiatric services is essential. As the population ages there will be a need for a greater number of support staff, such as psychiatric nurses and social workers, good quality respite facilities, ongoing support utilizing both the statutory and the voluntary sectors, and a recognition of the needs of the carers involved. Multidisciplinary specialist investigation units will be needed with memory clinics, inpatient investigation beds and support facilities. Specific treatments may be developed that will arrest or even reverse the progression of dementia. As depression results from an interaction of many variables, including intrinsic biological susceptibility to the condition, a future with improved income and living conditions, and better attention to prevention of disability, may see the incidence of depression decreasing.

Falling and mobility problems

Specialist-staffed falls clinics and rehabilitation services should be provided. Patients who fall need proper assessment and management. Many of the hospital patients who have fallen are not under the care of the geriatric medical services, they are under the care of orthopaedic teams. Good liaison between the two teams is essential so that the consequence of the fall (i.e. the fracture) is treated with reference to the reason for the fall. It is important to distinguish between basically well elderly people who suffer an accidental fall, usually out in the street, and the housebound frail, possibly sick, elderly people for whom the fall is a symptom of underlying disease.

Many elderly people present to a casualty department having fallen. Unless they have sustained obvious injury they are usually discharged with little thought and with no follow-up. Such people should be reviewed at home, possibly by a trained nurse or health visitor to try to assess whether or not they require any further investigation in a specific falls clinic or at a day hospital.

Patients who fall following a dizzy spell or syncope are particularly important, and the diagnostic yield if they are properly investigated, is high (McIntosh, Da Costa and Kenny,

1993). Even if a cause cannot be found, staff and patients should adopt a therapeutic approach to falls. With proper multidisciplinary assessment and advice, patients can be taught how to avoid and respond to falls in the future.

Stroke

Historically stroke illness was the 'poor relation' of medical conditions. Increasingly attention has been given to all aspects of treatment.

Prevention

Doctors and patients are increasingly aware of the benefits of preventive approaches, e.g. treating hypertension and the resultant demonstrable decrease in the incidence of stroke. Initiatives to encourage more exercise and cessation of smoking should have a similar effect on the incidence of the condition.

Acute management

There is as yet no consensus on the acute management of stroke. Trials are ongoing, looking at the use of aspirin and heparin. In future, we may well routinely admit patients to units analogous to coronary care units to provide the optimal management in the first few hours after a stroke, with particular attention to swallowing, nutrition, control of blood pressure, prevention of infection and antithrombotic therapy.

Rehabilitation

Trials that compared stroke units with general ward care have suggested that the outcome is better on designated stroke units (Langhorne *et al.*, 1993). It is not yet clear what particular components of such units produce the benefit. It may simply be that the therapy, nursing and medical staff are interested and dedicated to stroke care so the results they produce are better.

Incontinence

Incontinence of urine is a frequent problem in elderly patients that may not have been recognized by health and social service agencies, partly because patients are often reluctant

---

Practice points in stroke care
- Prevention
- Acute management
- Rehabilitation

to admit to it, but also because health professionals may not specifically ask. Future efforts should be targeted at reducing the stigma associated with the symptom, increasing the public's awareness of the potential for treatment, and educating doctors about the logical ways of approaching the problems. Management by teaching regimes such as pelvic floor exercises or bladder retraining, depending on the problem, is simple, and many patients can be successfully managed without recourse to full investigation. Most management will be dictated by the history, which will indicate whether the problem is stress incontinence or an urge incontinence that is likely to be due to detrusor instability. However, if the history is not conclusive, urodynamic investigation is required.

QUALITY AND LONG-TERM CARE

Physicians with experience in geriatric medicine should have a lead role in assessing and managing frail elderly patients and in deciding appropriate placement. Clearly this will require co-ordination with primary care teams and social services. Units within hospitals should provide a co-ordinated approach to the assessment of needs for residential and nursing care, perhaps on a day care basis. This might be part of an existing day hospital, or it might be that patients are booked in for a short stay in specific hospital beds for the purpose. Wherever elderly people are cared for it is essential that the staff should have adequate training. Research in our departments has shown that multiply handicapped frail elderly people can be cared for in personalized accommodation (Millard, 1991b). In the next century we expect this standard to be the rule not the exception.

Around the world there is considerable debate about the structure of long-term care for elderly people. Although it may be difficult to predict the exact style of future geriatric services, there are certain skills that must characterize our care. We must take full responsibility for our patient care. We must develop and use a wide knowledge base and practice in a spirit of service with a willingness to experiment. Medical leadership skills must also be developed and exercised within the multidisciplinary team if the various aspects of patient care are to be properly co-ordinated. Finally, we must ensure that physicians looking after elderly people in future are fully trained in these areas if we are in fact to provide elderly people with the care they deserve.

REFERENCES

Bagnall, W.E., Datta, S., Knox, J. and Horrocks, P. (1973) Geriatric medicine in Hull: a comprehensive service. *British Medical Journal*, **ii**, 102–4.

Carpenter, G.I. and Demopoulos, G.R. (1990) Screening the elderly in the community. *British Medical Journal*, **300**, 1258.

Chapuy, M.C., Arlot, M.E., Duboet, F. *et al.* (1992) Vitamin D3 + calcium to prevent hip fractures in elderly women. *New England Journal of Medicine*, **327**, 1637–42.

Feldstein, M.S. (1964) Effects of differences in hospital bed scarcity on type of use. *British Medical Journal*, **ii**, 561–5.

Grimley-Evans, J. (1994) High hopes for geriatrics – a view from the top. *Journal of the Royal College of Physicians*, **28**, 392–3.

Grundy, E. and Arie, T. (1984) Institutionalization and the elderly: international comparisons. *Age and Ageing*, **13**, 129–37.

Harrison, G.W. and Millard, P.H. (1991) Balancing acute and long term care: the mathematics of throughput in departments of geriatric medicine. *Methods of Information in Medicine*, **30**, 221–8.

Hodkinson, H.M. and Jeffreys, P.M. (1972) Making hospital geriatrics work. *British Medical Journal*, **4**, 536–9.

Horrocks, P. (1986) The components of a comprehensive district health service for elderly people – a personal view. *Age and Ageing*, **15**, 321–42.

House of Lords (1994) *Report of the select committee on medical ethics*, **volume I**, HMSO, London.

Irvine, V., McClean, S. and Millard, P.H. (1994) Stochastic models for geriatric in-patient behaviour. *IMA Journal of Mathematics Applied in Medicine and Biology*, **11**, 207–16.

Langhorne, P., Williams, B.O., Gilchrist, W. and Howie, K. (1993) Do stroke units save lives? *The Lancet*, **342**, 395–8.

MacLennan, W.J. (1990) Screening elderly patients: a task well suited to health visitors. *British Medical Journal*, **300**, 694–5.

McClean, S.I. (1994) Modelling and simulation for health care systems, in *Modelling hospital resource use: a different approach to the planning and control of health care systems* (eds P.H. Millard and S.I. McClean), Royal Society of Medicine, London.

McClean, S. and Millard, P.H. (1993) Modelling in-patient bed usage behaviour in a department of geriatric medicine. *Methods of Information in Medicine*, **32**, 79–81.

McIntosh, S., Da Costa, D. and Kenny, R.A. (1993) Outcomes of an integrated approach to the investigation of dizziness, falls and syncope in elderly patients referred to a syncope clinic. *Age and Ageing*, **22**, 53–8.

McMurdo, M.E.T. and Rennie, L. (1993) A controlled trial of exercise by residents of old people's homes. *Age and Ageing*, **22**, 11–15.

Millard, P.H. (1989) Geriatric medicine: a new method of measuring bed usage and a theory for planning. MD thesis, University of London.

Millard, P.H. (1991a) A case for the development of departments of gerocomy in all district general hospitals. *Journal of the Royal Society of Medicine*, **84**, 731–3.

Millard, P.H. (1991b) The Bolingbroke Hospital long-term care project, in *Care of the long-stay elderly patient* (ed. M.J. Denham), 2nd edn, Chapman & Hall, London, pp. 283–98.

Millard, P.H. (1992) Throughput in a department of geriatric medicine: a problem of time, space and behaviour. *Health Trends*, **24**, 20–4.

Millard, P.H. (1994) Meeting the needs of an ageing population. *Proceedings of the Royal College of Physicians of Edinburgh*, **24**, 187–96.

Millard, P.H., McClean, S.I. (eds) (1994) *Modelling hospital resource use: a different approach to the planning and control of health care systems*, London: Royal Society of Medicine Press.

Millard, P.H. McClean, S.I. (eds) (1996) *Go with the Flow: a systems approach to healthcare planning*, Royal Society of Medicine Press.

Millard Associates (1993) *BOMPS: the bed occupancy management and planning system*, St George's Hospital Medical School http://www.sghms.ac.uk/gm/index htm.

Pfeiffer, E. (1985) Some basic principles of working with older patients. *Journal of the American Geriatrics Society*, **33**, 44–7.

Roebothan, B.V. and Chandra, R.K. (1994) Relationship between nutritional status and immune function of elderly people. *Age and Ageing*, **23**, 49–53.

Royal College of Physicians of London (1994) *Ensuring equity and quality of care for elderly people. The interface between geriatric medicine and general (internal) medicine*, Royal College of Physicians, London.

Silver, C.P. and Zuberi, S.J. (1965) Prognosis of patients admitted to a geriatric unit. *Gerontologia Clinica*, **7**, 348–57.

Warren, M.W. (1943) Care of the chronic sick: a case for treating the chronic sick in blocks in a general hospital. *British Medical Journal*, **ii**, 822–3.

Yates, J. (1982) *Hospital beds: a problem for diagnosis and management*, William Heinemann, London.

Appendix
Useful addresses

Advice Services Alliance
13 Stockwell Road
London SW9 9AU
Tel: 0171-274 1878

Age Concern England
Astral House
1268 London Road
London SW16 4ER
Tel: 0181-679 8000

Age Concern Scotland
54a Fountainbridge
Edinburgh EH3 9PT
Tel: 0131-467 7118

Alzheimer's Disease Society
Gordon House
10 Greencoat Place
London SW1P 1PH
Tel: 0171-306 0606

Arthritis and Rheumatism Council
PO Box 177
Chesterfield
Derbyshire S41 7TQ
Tel: 01246-558033

Association of Chartered Physiotherapists with a Special Interest in Elderly People
c/o Chartered Society of Physiotherapy
15 Bedford Row
London WC1R 4ED
Tel: 0171-242 1941

Association of Continence Advisers
2 Doughty Street
London WC1N 2PH
Tel: 0171-404 6821

Association of Directors of Social Services
c/o Social Services Central Offices
County Hall
Northallerton DK7 8DD
Tel: 01609-770661

Audit Commission
1 Vincent Square
London SW1P 2PF
Tel: 0171-828 1212

British Association of Social Workers
16 Kent Street
Birmingham B5 6RD
Tel: 0121-622 3911

British College of Occupational Therapists
6–8 Marshalsea Road
London SE1 1HL
Tel: 0171-357 6480

British Diabetic Association
10 Queen Anne Street
London W1M 0BD
Tel: 0171-323 1531

British Dietetic Association
7th Floor
Elizabeth House
22 Suffolk Street
Queensway
Birmingham B1 1LS
Tel: 0121-643 5483

British Geriatrics Society
1 St Andrew's Place
Regent's Park
London NW1 4LB
Tel: 0171-935 4004

British Medical Association
BMA House
Tavistock Square
London WC1H 9JP
Tel: 0171-387 4499

British Psychological Society
St Andrew's House
48 Princes Road East
Leicester LE1 7DR
Tel: 01533-549568

British Society of Audiology
80 Briton Road
Reading RG6 1PS
Tel: 01734-660622

British Society of Hearing Therapists
The Hearing Centre
Yardley Green Unit
East Birmingham Hospital
Birmingham B9 5PX
Tel: 0121-766 6611 ext 2556

British Society of Rheumatology
3 St Andrew's Place
London NW1 4LE
Tel: 0171-224 3739

Carers' National Association
29 Chilworth Mews
London W2 3RG
Tel: 0171-490 8818

Central Council for Education and Training in Social Work
Derbyshire House
St Chad's Street
London WC1H 8AD
Tel: 0171-278 2455

Centre for Environmental Studies in Ageing
Ladbroke House
62–66 Highbury Grove
London N5 2AD
Tel: 0171-753 5038

Centre for Policy on Ageing
25–31 Ironmonger Row
London EC1V 3PQ
Tel: 0171-253 1787

Chartered Society of Physiotherapy
14 Bedford Row
London WC1R 4ED
Tel: 0171-242 1941

Citizens' Advocacy, Information and Training
Leroy House
436 Essex Road
London N1 3UP
Tel: 0171-359 8289

College of Occupational Therapists
6 Marshalsea Road
London SE1 1HL
Tel: 0171-357 6480

College of Speech and Language Therapists
7 Bath Place
Rivington Street
London EC2A 3TR
Tel: 0171-613 3855

Community and District Nursing Association (UK)
Thames Valley University
8 University House
Ealing Green
London W5 5ED
Tel: 0181-231 2776

Counsel and Care for the Elderly
Twyman House
16 Bonny Street
London NW1 9PG
Tel: 0171-485 1550

Crossroads Caring for Carers
10 Regent Place
Rugby
CV21 2PN
Tel: 01788 573653

Department of Health
Skipton House
80 London Road
London SE1 6LW
Tel: 0171-972 2000

Department of Health, Social Services Inspectorate
Wellington House
133–155 Waterloo Road
London SE1 8UG
Tel: 0171-407 5522

Disabled Living Foundation
380–384 Harrow Road
London W9 2HL
Tel: 0171-289 6111

Eurolink Age
1268 London Road
London SW16 4ER
Tel: 0181-679 8000

Health Education Authority
Hamilton House
Mabledon Place
London WC1A 9TY
Tel: 0171-383 3833

Hearing Concern
7–11 Armstrong Road
London W3 7JL
Tel: 0181-743 1110

Help the Aged
16–18 St. James's Walk
London EC1R 0BE
Tel: 0171 253 0253

Institute of Health Service Managers
39 Chalton Street
London NW1 1JD
Tel: 0171 388 2626

King Edward's Hospital Fund
14 Palace Court
London W2 4HT
Tel: 0171-727 0581

King's Fund Centre
11–13 Cavendish Square
London W1M 0AN
Tel: 0171-307 2400

King's Fund Centre Mail Order
BEBC Distribution
15 Albion Close
Parkstone
Poole BH12 3LL
Tel: 0800 262260 (freephone)

MIND (National Association for Mental Health)
Granta House
15–19 Broadway
Stratford
London E15 4BQ
Tel: 0181-519 2122

National Association of Health Authorities and Trusts
Birmingham Research Park
Vincent Drive
Birmingham B15 2SQ
Tel: 0121-471 4444

**National Council for Hospice and Specialist Palliative Care
Services**
59 Bryanston Street
London W1A 2AZ
Tel: 0171-611 1153

National Council for Voluntary Organizations
Regent's Wharf
8 All Saints Street
London N1 9RL
Tel: 0171-713 6161

National Information Forum
380–384 Harrow Road
London W9 2HU
Tel: 0171-289 1670

National Institute for Social Work
5–7 Tavistock Place
London WC1H 9SN
Tel: 0171-387 9681

NHS Executive Headquarters
Quarry House, Quarry Hill
Leeds LS2 7UE
Tel: 0113 2545205

Parkinson's Disease Society
36 Portland Place
London W1N 3DG
Tel: 0171-383 3513

Prince of Wales' Advisory Group on Disability
8 Bedford Road
London WC1R 4BU
Tel: 0171-430 0558

Psychologists' Special Interest Group in the Elderly (Special Interest Group of the Division of Clinical Psychology of the British Psychological Society)
Department of Clinical Psychology
Parkhead Hospital
81 Salamanca Street
Glasgow G31 5BA
Tel: 0141-211 8300

Research into Ageing
Baird House
15–17 St Cross Street
London EC1N 8UN
Tel: 0171 404 6878

Royal Association for Disability and Rehabilitation
25 Mortimer Street
London W1N 8AB
Tel: 0171-250 3222

Royal College of General Practitioners
14 Princes Gate
London SW7 1PU
Tel: 0171-581 3232

Royal College of Nursing of the UK
20 Cavendish Square
London W1M 9AE
Tel: 0171-409 3333

Royal College of Physicians, London
11 St Andrew's Place
London NW1 4LE
Tel: 0171-935 1174

Royal College of Physicians, Edinburgh
9 Queen Street
Edinburgh EH2 WQ
Tel: 0131-225 7324

Royal College of Physicians and Surgeons, Glasgow
232–242 St Vincent Street
Glasgow, G2 5RJ
Tel: 0141-221 6072

Royal College of Psychiatrists
17 Belgrave Square
London SW1X 8PG
Tel: 0171-235 2351

Royal National Institute for the Blind
247 Great Portland Street
London W1N 6AA
Tel: 0171-388 1266

Royal National Institute for Deaf People
19–23 Featherstone Street
London EC1Y 8SL
Tel: 0171-296 8000

Royal Pharmaceutical Society of Great Britain
1 Lambeth High Street
London SE1 7JR
Tel: 0171-735 9141

Scottish Action on Dementia
8 Hill Street
Edinburgh EH2 3JZ
Tel: 0131-220 4886

Scottish Office Social Work Services Group
43 Jeffrey Street
Edinburgh EH1 1DN
Tel: 0131-556 8400

Social Care Association
23A Victoria Road
Surbiton KT6 4JZ
Tel: 0181-390 4639

Society of Chiropodists
53 Welbeck Street
London W1H 7HE
Tel: 0171-486 3381

Stroke Association
Tavistock House North
Tavistock Square
London WC1H 9JE
Tel: 0171-490 7999

The Volunteer Centre UK
Carriage Road
129 Eversholt Street
London NW1 1BU
Tel: 0171-388 9888

**UK Central Council for Nursing, Midwifery and Health
  Visitors**
23 Portland Place
London W1N 3AF
Tel: 0171-637 7181

UK Home Care Association
206 Worple Road
London SW20 8PN
Tel: 0181-946 8202

Index